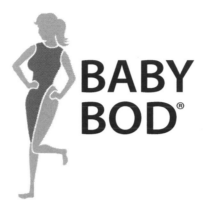

BABY BOD®

TURN FLAB TO FAB IN 12 WEEKS FLAT

A Groundbreaking Program
for Pregnant and Postpartum Women

Marianne Ryan, PT, OCS

This book is intended as a reference volume only, not as a medical manual. The information given here is designed to help you make informed decisions about your health. It is not intended as a substitute for any treatment that may have been prescribed by your doctor, midwife, or physical therapist. If you suspect that you have a medical problem, I urge you to seek competent medical help.

Printed in the United States of America

Editor: Deborah Grandinetti
Illustrations by M. Rusdiato
Illustration Editor: Garegin Nalbandian
Cover Design: Laurie Binder
Book Design: Robert Marcus Graphics

Library of Congress Cataloging-in-Publication Data
2014922125

ISBN 978-0-9890351-0-1

Table of Contents

Praise for Baby Bod®

*"It is time for women to consider each stage of healing post-birth and take the time needed for full recovery. **Baby Bod**® will help women who are still postnatal many years later, as well as new mums, make the journey to recovery from pregnancy and childbirth."*

— **Dianne Edmonds**, Director and Founder of The Pregnancy Centre, Physiotherapist, Personal Trainer

*"**Baby Bod**® is a must-read not just for moms, but for all women suffering the real effects of improper use of muscles. This well-written, easy-to-read book challenges readers to change their paradigms and think about a team approach to women's care. The team can include the physiotherapist, physical therapist, and OB-GYN. The author uses solid research to back up her teaching. Reading this book with an open mind can result in, well . . . results!"*

— **Dr. LaKeischa Webb McMillan, OB-GYN** and mother of two

"An excellent and comprehensive guide for expectant and new mums on how to safely maintain and regain correct body alignment and core and pelvic floor strength throughout the often confusing stages of body changes they experience during pregnancy and early motherhood."

— **Fiona Rogers BPhty GD ExSpSc APAM**
Pelvic Floor Physiotherapist
Owner, www.pelvicfloorexercise.com.au

*"I am thrilled to have this resource to share with mothers and birth professionals that finally bridges the gap between medical care and fitness advice. Birth professionals will find this book helpful when teaching their clients how to protect their bodies with correct body mechanics. This is a sound and safe guide to start building the pelvic floor and core muscles right after birth. Getting back in shape after childbirth is about more than just looking our best. Strengthening these muscles correctly will positively affect our future pregnancies, consequent births, sexual health, and even help prevent prolapse during menopause. **Baby Bod**® is grounded in evidence-based solutions that address anatomy and physiology in the most holistic way. Best yet, the book is brilliantly designed to guide you*

*through chapters depending on where you are – because none of us have precious time to waste, especially while caring for a newborn. I highly recommend all women read **Baby Bod**®, even before they give birth, so that they are well informed and ready to celebrate their own **Baby Bod**® when the time comes."*

— **Tara Brooke CD (DTI)**, Co-founder, Doula Trainings International
Doula and New Parent Consultant and mother of three

*"Until now, pregnant women, new moms, and clinicians have not had an accessible reference book that covers everything they need to know before and after delivering that bundle of joy. **Baby Bod**® is that book. In **Baby Bod**®, Marianne Ryan, PT, OCS synthesizes an impressive array of literature into a reader-friendly format that covers maternal health and wellbeing, self-care tips, and progressive exercises. Her information is well-presented and thoughtfully curated. She offers knowledge acquired from her own clinical and personal experience as well as the latest evidence-based research to back it up. What a great resource for any new or experienced mom who is interested in re-shaping her mind and body before and after birth. I only wish I had this book when I delivered my two sons, but I look forward to offering this book to my patients and friends."*

— **Stacy Barrows, PT, DPT, GCFP, PMA®-CPT**
Inventor of the Smartroller®, Author of the Smartroller Guide to
Optimal Movement / owner of Century City Physical Therapy, Inc.

"This is a reassuring and comprehensive guide for mothers at every stage of life who want to feel good in their bodies. Ryan clearly and thoroughly explains how pregnancy affects a woman's body, and she offers insightful tips on how to strengthen it from head to toe."

— **Rachel Rabkin Peachman**, Journalist

*"**Baby Bod**® is an excellent resource for Moms of any age! This is a well-referenced, evidence-based guide on how to prevent, heal or rehab the core at any age or stage of the game. The information is delivered in a practical manner that presents a useful guide for anyone to follow. This book will have a prominent place in my clinic and will be a successful tool for my wellness and rehab clients."*

— **Susan C. Clinton PT DScPT OCS WCS COMT FAAOMPT**
Co-Owner of Embody Physiotherapy & Wellness, LLC

"This book is a game changer! Marianne Ryan has used her experience as a mother and a leading Women's Health Physical Therapist to develop a programme suitable for mums to be, and new and experienced mums. Physical Therapists and health professionals looking after these women will benefit from it also. It will allow mums to recognize and manage the key conditions like diastasis, pelvic girdle pain, bladder leakage and prolapse. Read it, follow the program, and get yourself back to full health and fitness."

— **Gerard Greene MSc** (Manip Physio) Specialist Musculoskeletal Physical Therapist, Educator & Co-founder, Women's Health Physio Facebook group.

"Marianne goes where no woman has gone before. She answers questions that have not been answered for generations for first time (and many time) moms. **Baby Bod**® has the formula you need to get your body back, perhaps even better than before your pregnancy. **Baby Bod**® is the 'Dr. Spock' book for moms that we have all been waiting for."

— **Mark Alyn**, Host, Late Night Health Radio

"**Baby Bod**® explains the musculoskeletal effects of pregnancy and labor in a way that all patients will understand. Whether you are pregnant for the first time or have had multiple children, it's an important read for all!"

— **Jaclyn H. Bonder, MD**, Medical Director, Women's Health Rehabilitation and Assistant Professor, Weill Cornell Medical College

"I loved reading **Baby Bod**®. Ryan draws together the complexities of a woman's body after childbirth in a way that explains, reassures, and provides sensible, evidence-informed advice based on her long experience in women's health physical therapy.

The **Baby Bod**® exercise programme is excellent. I tried all the exercises and found the explanations and illustrations very reader-friendly. The book builds up the knowledge needed to do the exercises and also explains why they are so important after having a baby, whether immediately after birth, or many years later. The phrase "once postpartum, always post-partum" will resonate for many women.

This is a perfect gift for friends, sisters, daughters, mothers, and grandmothers."

— **Emma Stokes**, Physiotherapist Vice President, World Confederation for Physical Therapy

Acknowledgments

You know the saying, "It takes a village?" Well, that was true for **BabyBod**®, too.

My thanks go, first of all, to all the female physical therapy clients who graced my Manhattan practice over the past 30 years. Thank you for trusting me as your therapist and for allowing me to grow as a professional.

I also want to say thank you to Dr. Anne Carlon, a talented and caring doctor. Anne, thank you for entrusting me with the many patients you've referred over the past 25 years. And thank you for your enthusiastic "yes" when I asked you to write the foreword to this book. It's absolutely beautiful.

I also want to acknowledge the many bright and caring physical therapists and physiotherapists who went out of their way to be helpful during the three years it took to write this book. This is a long list so I won't be able to name everyone, but I do want to single out Lila Bartkowski Abbate, Stacy Barrows, Sue Croft, Dianne Edmonds, Ginger Gardner, Debbie Goetz, Gerard Greene, Sandy Hilton, Diane Lee, Antony Lo, Elaine Miller, Fiona Rodgers, and Julie Wiebe. You have all been so generous and encouraging, sharing research articles and your advice and clinical expertise. An especially big thank you to Antony Lo for all the hours you spent reviewing the core muscle and stability system chapters and discussing them with me over Skype.

Special thanks to my co-worker and schoolmate, Barbara Carbone, a terrific physical therapist. Barbara, the model for many of the exercise illustrations in the book, suffered through at least five photo sessions so that we could get these just right. Some sessions were particularly arduous; she held uncomfortable poses for a long time so we could capture just the right angle. For that, Barbara, I am endlessly grateful. Mohammad Rusdianto, a fabulous graphic artist, converted these photos into drawings. A big thank you, Mohammad, for all your wonderful illustrations. Gargin Nalbandian did a wonderful job of editing these illustrations, thank you Gargin.

Much gratitude also to my terrific editor, Deborah Grandinetti. Her calming resolve was the perfect match for my "energetic" personality. We made a great team, and I miss our weekly talks. We became friends, which was a wonderful surprise and an added bonus to writing this book. Deborah, without you, this book would not have been completed. Thanks for believing in this project and me all the way through, and for all your great work figuring out how to organize everything.

I also want to thank Jeanette Lopez for your painstaking work in organizing and formatting the endnotes and footnotes, a tedious task for sure. Thanks to your keen organizational skills, Jeannette, I am confident that book properly cites all the research and acknowledges all the people who generously shared clinical tips.

Thanks also go to the graphic artists—Laurie Binder, and Robert Marcus—for their work converting the manuscript and illustrations into a book. I especially want to acknowledge Laurie for her wonderful book cover and interior design. Laurie, I love it!

Finally, a huge thank you to my family! My husband, Colin, was very patient and gave me enough space to focus on writing. Colin read the manuscript at least five or six times to make sure it was free of typos and other mistakes. He also took over some household chores and commandeered the move into a new apartment so I could keep on top of my demanding schedule. Colin, thank you for *everything*! And much thanks to my two daughters, Caitlyn and Maggie, for their enthusiastic support over the life of this project. Caitlyn and Maggie, I am especially grateful for your help in making the client stories in this book more enjoyable and less "nerdy!"

* * *

Foreword

In thirty years of practice, I have been privileged to help thousands of women safely deliver healthy babies. During the months of pregnancy, continuous attention is lavished, rightfully, on every aspect of the mother and baby's health. After delivery, however, most of the care is directed to the baby, or to the unique forms of support that only a mother can provide, such as breastfeeding. Attention to helping mothers themselves restore their physical state has been sadly lacking.

This is in part due to the common expectation that most mothers will recover quickly from the birth experience and will be ready to return to a normal life within a few weeks. While it is true that medical advances have led to a decrease in the most severe complications of childbirth such as hemorrhage and sepsis, modern women need no longer be satisfied simply with surviving pregnancy without serious complications. They should be able to enjoy pregnancy, delivery and motherhood as a uniquely positive experience. A prolonged period of recovery after childbirth, leaving a mother weaker and in poorer physical shape than before she became pregnant, inevitably diminishes the quality of that experience. Women should be able to prevent or address other potential consequences of childbirth, such as pain, weakness, incontinence, and prolapse.

Marianne Ryan's book, **Baby Bod**®, directly and comprehensively addresses the steps that any woman can take during pregnancy, after childbirth and even years later to quickly and conveniently restore her physical strength to the same condition it was before pregnancy.

A recognized expert in the fields of physical fitness and physical therapy, author Marianne Ryan combines 30 years of clinical experience in the treatment of problems of the spine and pelvis with a distinguished record as an educator at the Columbia University Nurse Midwifery Programs, alongside many other achievements in the academic and public education are acknowledgments. Ms. Ryan was inspired to write this book not only by her professional experience as a physical therapist, but also by her own personal experiences with childbirth. After having two children of her own, she had been unable to find, among the countless self-help books for new mothers, one that addressed the importance of recovering physical fitness while providing practical guidelines to achieve that coveted goal.

The recommendations contained in this book are based on strong clinical evidence as well as the evaluation of over one hundred new mothers treated by Ms. Ryan. Its instructions are written in a smooth, discursive style which most women will be able to follow comfortably. Its clear explanations of basic anatomy make the program entirely logical and easy to comprehend.

The circumstances of each delivery are unique. For example, women may have uncomplicated vaginal births, perineal lacerations or cesarean sections. **Baby Bod**® addresses this range of possibilities and provides specific advice related to each of these situations so as to allow every mother the opportunity to regain her physical fitness. Ms. Ryan understands that the life of a new mother is fragmented and cannot necessarily conform to a predictable schedule. The exercises described in her book can be spread throughout the day, to accommodate the unique needs of mother and baby. Also included are comprehensive instructions on the correct ways to perform daily activities, as well as suggestions regarding both "baby" gear and "mommy" gear.

While the book is primarily directed at women who have already delivered, many of the recommended exercises and activities can be started during pregnancy to maintain the best physical condition at the time of delivery. Equally important, women who have delivered years earlier can use this program to address the long-term physical consequences of childbirth.

Ms. Ryan wisely recognizes that not all problems are amenable to self-help. Sometimes it is necessary to consult a health professional, and her book offers reasonable guidelines to assist new mothers in determining when medical assistance is needed. The book includes useful self-assessment checklists and worksheets that can be given to healthcare providers, if necessary, to help determine clinical problems before they become more troublesome.

As an obstetrician/gynecologist (and as a mother), I'm delighted to have witnessed an increase in the attention paid to the physical recovery of postpartum women postpartum. At last there is a practical and effective approach for women to take, one which is thoroughly and clearly explained in this essential book.

Anne T. Carlon, MD
Assistant Attending Obstetrician and Gynecologist
New York Presbyterian Hospital
New York, New York

Introduction

A woman's body is a wonderful instrument, something never more apparent than when she becomes pregnant. In response to the new life growing within her, her own body begins to change in ways she could not have imagined. Everything happens on cue. Breasts grow and eventually become milk machines, that flat tummy gradually morphs into a mama belly, and ligaments that once held muscle and bone securely loosen so that the pelvic bones can move apart enough to allow the baby's head enough space to pass through the birth canal.

And then, the baby is born, launching the woman into the strange new land called Motherhood.

At some point afterward, as the new mom catches a glimpse of her physical metamorphosis in the mirror, she can't help but ask herself:

"What the $#@& happened to my body? How soon will it take to get my pre-pregnancy body back? I will be able to get the old one back, right?"

* * *

Having a baby isn't all sunshine and roses. Pregnancy and childbirth can be an extremely exciting time in a woman's life, yet also bring a long list of lingering physical challenges. That's right—I'm talking about a flabby "Mommy Tummy," leaky bladder, and lower back pain, just to name a few. A lot of new moms simply aren't comfortable discussing these changes, even with their doctors.

That's part of the problem. The other part: While most women receive top-notch care during pregnancy and delivery, the majority of healthcare professionals often forget to address the needs of the woman behind that belly, after she gives birth. As a culture, we seem to have the attitude that the physical strains placed on a woman's body as a result of childbirth are temporary and that everything will somehow magically revert back to normal "over time."

This is not true.

These changes can lead to lifelong problems—some of them very serious.

This happens far more often than it should—in large part because a few days after delivery the only postpartum care most women receive is *one* checkup six weeks after the blessed event. If you have no major complications and you don't mention pain or incontinence at that time, you're on your own. You're given a pat on the back for a job well done, a "green light" to resume all normal activities, and a piece of paper telling you how to do Kegel exercises. Then off you go. Typically, that's all the postnatal care you'll get. Period. End of story.

From my personal experience and my perspective as a physical therapist, it's *crazy* to drop the ball after six short weeks. Six weeks leaves just enough time—if that—for the *first* stage of soft tissue to heal. It can take several months or more for the abdominal and pelvic muscles to fully recover. (If you breastfeed, it takes more time, for reasons I will explain in depth in Chapter Five.) The postpartum body is especially vulnerable to injury at this time, which is why it's so important to know how to properly care for it.

I am one of the new breed of physical therapists who specialize in women's health and I am passionate about helping women overcome the often-overlooked postpartum issues I just described. I can relate well to other moms because I suffered from recurrent back pain and a leaky bladder for over two decades after giving birth to my two children. During the years that followed, I tried several different exercise programs and months of biofeedback. But nothing helped until I developed the **Baby Bod® Program**. I designed it to heal myself and help women like me *fully* recover from childbirth. It permanently resolved my problems and proved successful when tested on over 100 women. It's a revolutionary program because it bridges the gap between evidence-based medical science and fitness instruction.

* * *

It can be overwhelming enough to welcome a new baby into the world. Dealing with the physical after effects of childbirth while caring for a newborn can prove to be just too much, as I well know. With **Baby Bod**®, however, you don't have to accept these unwanted changes as the "new normal."

The **Baby Bod**® **Program** I share in this book is a gentle, effective solution that will help you restore your body from the inside out. It's conveniently DIY, so you can do it on your schedule. You can start it while you are pregnant, one day after delivery, or even years after becoming a mother—and still get great results. In the book, I will take you through a simple step-by-step recovery program. You'll learn why your body doesn't just "snap back together" after childbirth, what you can do to prevent injuries, and how to recover your pre-pregnancy shape. Best of all, the program will help you *"Turn Flab to Fab in 12 weeks Flat."*

* * *

The Baby Bod® Program will teach you how to:

- flatten that "Mommy Tummy"
- relieve pain
- prevent injuries
- care for your new baby without developing aches and pains, and
- return to sports safely.

HOW TO USE THE BOOK

Because the **Baby Bod® Program** is for women at different stages on the birth continuum, I've organized the book so that you only need to read the material that pertains to you. Chapter One addresses the pregnant mom; Chapter Two, the new mom; and Chapter Three, the experienced mom. Start with the chapter that's meant for you, then skip to Chapter Four and read straight through Chapter Seven.

These middle chapters will teach you what you need to know to make the best use of the program and to prevent yourself from sustaining the kind of injury that will stall your recovery. (As an added bonus, you can also use this knowledge to evaluate the suitability of other fitness programs that interest you.) Please read all of those chapters first; DO NOT go straight to the exercise chapters.

Chapters Eight and Nine offer great self-care advice you can use as soon as you have the baby. Read Chapter Eight if you plan to have—or have had—a vaginal birth; read Chapter Nine if you plan to have—or have had—a Cesarean birth.

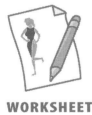

WORKSHEET

Worksheets

I have provided worksheets so that you can record your progress on the self-assessment tests in these chapters. (Look for the worksheet logo.) You'll find the worksheets in Appendix A in the back of the book. You'll want to make a copy of these pages so that they're available to bring with you the next time you visit your doctor, midwife, or physical therapist.

The exercise program kicks off with a chapter on exercise guidelines in Chapter Ten. The exercise component has a preliminary and advanced phase. You'll find the **Preliminary Phase Exercises** in Chapters Eleven to Fourteen, and the **Advanced Strengthening Exercises** in Chapter Fifteen. (Charts that summarize the exercises can be found in the appendices.)

The last two chapters of the book help you bring the program into your everyday life. Chapter Sixteen explains how to choose nursery room furniture and other baby gear that supports rather than strains your body. (If you're buying baby things now, you may want to read that chapter first). Chapter Seventeen teaches you how to apply what you've learned to everyday movements, such as reaching down to diaper the baby. If you do what I suggest, you'll not only prevent common back and neck injuries, but get that flat tummy even faster!

Enough talk. Pregnant women, are you ready for a safe and effective workout that will put your body into the best possible shape for childbirth? Postpartum moms, are you ready to turn flab to fab in 12 weeks flat?

Then turn the page and let's get started!!!

CHAPTER ONE

Baby Bod® During Pregnancy: For the Mommies-to-Be Among Our Readers

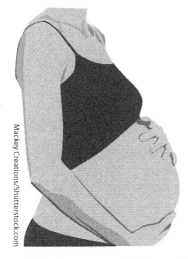

Mackey Creations/Shutterstock.com

If you've gotten hold of this book while you're still pregnant, I applaud you on your foresight. If you were given this book as a shower gift, consider yourself lucky indeed. That's because you're in the best position to get the most out of it. Not only can you start using this book now, I *urge you* to do so for a few good reasons:

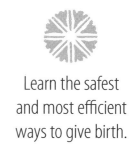

Learn the safest and most efficient ways to give birth.

1. Studies have shown many *positive benefits of exercise during pregnancy.* The American College of Obstetrics and Gynecology guidelines state "in the absence of either medical or obstetrical complications, 30 minutes or more of moderate exercise on most, if not all, days of the week is recommended for pregnant women." [1] Exercises like the ones in the **Baby Bod®** program can reduce incontinence (urine leakage) during pregnancy. [2]

2. **It's good for the baby.** Exercising while you are pregnant increases the blood flowing to the baby's brain and may help to make your baby smarter! [3]

3. **Learning the Baby Bod® exercises prior to your delivery** will make it easier for you to start them up again soon after you've

given birth—and that **will give you a jump on your recovery after childbirth.** You have a bit more "me time" now than you will have after you give birth, so it will be easier for you to learn at your own pace. You'll do a week of the **Preliminary Phase Exercises** and then move on to the **Advanced Phase Exercises**—unless you have been advised not to exercise by your health care professional.

4. The more advanced exercises **will put your body in the best shape possible to handle the rigors of labor and delivery.**[A] Let me assure you that the exercises in both phases of the **Baby Bod® Program** are absolutely safe for you up until the day you deliver. (There are a few exercises I'll ask you to skip until after you give birth, but these are very clearly marked.) Then you'll resume the **Preliminary Phase Exercises** a day or so after you give birth.

5. You can save yourself and your body a lot of trouble by **learning about the safest and most efficient ways to give birth,** which I discuss below. This will optimize your birthing experience.

6. **You can spare your back and neck many aches and pains—** and teach your partner to do the same—**by reading and acting on my advice on how to create an ergonomic nursery** and how to use good body mechanics during exercise and your everyday activities. I will cover these topics in depth throughout the book.

7. **You will learn what to pack in your overnight bag to make yourself more comfortable immediately after birth.** You can find this list later on in this chapter. It would also be good for you to read about the various kinds of external support garments and belts that can help speed healing. You'll find this information in Chapters Eight and Nine.[B] If you plan to use any of these garments,

---

[A] If any exercise causes pain, stop doing it and wait until after you've given birth to resume that exercise.

[B] Both chapters provide you with self-care advice you can use immediately after you have your baby. If you expect to give birth vaginally, see Chapter 8. If you plan to have a C-section, please see Chapter 9.

it would be helpful to buy them now so you'll have them right after you give birth.

I hope I've convinced you!

These days, women are a lot more active during pregnancy. Most of my pregnant clients tell me, "I'm going to work until my water breaks." I think it's good for women to remain active and to exercise throughout their pregnancy. If you plan to do this, just remember that not all exercise is equal. If you're pregnant, you want to avoid—or at least reduce the intensity of—any sports or activities that require you to jump or balance on one leg, as well as any that might jar the body. This is especially important during the last trimester.

In my mind, the most ideal exercises to do while you are pregnant are the **Baby Bod® exercises** in this book and low-impact cardio such as the elliptical machine and stationary bike. These will prepare you for your postpartum recovery in a way other exercise programs won't. Just avoid the exercises that ask you to lie on your back. Current guidelines suggest that pregnant woman should NOT exercise while lying on their backs after the first trimester.[4] To make sure you do not forget to stop when you reach your second trimester, I advise all pregnant women to not exercise while lying on their backs throughout the entire pregnancy. Don't worry—I will remind you when I give you the exercise instructions. Also, if you experience dizziness or pain while exercising, stop immediately and report it to your midwife or doctor.

There's just one exercise in the Preliminary Phase that will prove to be a challenge once you're in the later stages of your pregnancy: the **Baby Bod® Alignment Check**.[5] Here's the reason why it's a challenge: Eventually, the size of the baby will prevent you from bringing your rib cage over your pelvis, which is what I ask you to do. Don't worry about doing it perfectly; just do it the best you can without causing discomfort. But don't skip it!

* * *

Enough about the exercises! Here are five other things you should be thinking about as you prepare to deliver your baby:

Talk to Your ObGyn or Midwife about the Safest Birthing Practices[5]

There's no time like the present to talk to your physician or nurse midwife about the safest birthing practices. There have been some relatively new findings—new enough that your healthcare practitioners may not have caught onto them yet—that specific birthing practices can prevent common post-pregnancy complications, such as pelvic organ prolapse (POP for short.) This is a condition where organs such as the uterus or bowels slip down from their normal positions inside of the pelvis and lead to pelvic pain and incontinence (urine and fecal). I'll cover POP in more detail in Chapter Seven, but for now, I just want to make you aware that the wrong birthing techniques can put you at greater risk for developing this condition.

In general, the more strain placed on the pelvic floor during childbirth, the more a woman is at risk of developing POP and tearing in the pelvic floor and vagina. The right birthing techniques—which consider the amount of time a woman is allowed to labor, breathing techniques, and the type of birthing position she uses—can minimize that strain.[6]

Experts say that the key to preventing POP and pelvic floor tearing is giving women **enough time to labor** and **not** asking women to push **until they feel the urge to do so**.[6] (This might require as much as two hours for first-time moms.) In short, you should push when you feel a contraction. This allows the natural contractions of the uterus to "expel" the baby, rather than forcing the baby through a canal that has not been given enough of a chance to fully expand in preparation for childbirth.

Another thing to consider is **breathing techniques** used during labor and delivery. Did you know that holding your breath increases pressure in your belly and that this increased pressure pushes the pelvic organs downwards, which increases your risk of developing pelvic organ prolapse and/or of sustaining damage to your pelvic floor? "Breath holding" (holding your breath) also makes the deeper abdominal muscles work less efficiently at a time when they are needed most to help push your baby through the birth canal.

"**Purple pushing**," a common practice used in childbirth, is an example of a breath-holding technique that can be problematic; it too can lead to damage during childbirth. In "purple pushing," the expectant mom is asked to hold her breath and bear down for the count of ten while she is pushing the baby out. A better breathing technique for both the mother and the baby is to EXHALE while you push; this will encourage the abdominal muscles to work more efficiently to get that baby out.

Birthing positions can also influence whether a woman develops pelvic organ prolapse. Some positions will make it easier for the baby to pass down the birth canal and decrease the risk of injures and tears during delivery. The most common position is to have a woman lie on her back with her feet up in stirrups.

Guess what?

The hardest position to deliver in is lying on your back with your thighs rotated outwards (this is, when your knees are pointed outwards) and feet in stirrups. This is because the bones at the bottom of the pelvis actually move closer together in this position, rather than spreading out for delivery. Since the diameter of the birth canal is decreased in this position, the baby's head will place even more pressure on the vaginal walls and pelvic floor muscles during the delivery, which increases the risk of developing tears that can lead to pelvic organ prolapse later down the road. Yikes! (I delivered both of my kids in that position; no wonder I had to get two episiotomies!)

Positions that allow the thighs to internally rotate, with the knees slightly rotated *towards* each other, increase the diameter of the birth canal and decrease the risk of injury. Some examples of birthing positions that will accomplish this are side-lying and birthing while on your hands and knees.

Also consider choosing a position that encourages gravity to assist in delivery. Gravity-assisted positions such as standing and some modified squatting positions should help your baby pass down the birthing canal.

If you'd like to provide your ObGyn or midwife with a credible article published on this subject, I recommend getting your hands on a copy of "When and How to Push: Providing the Most Current Information about Second-Stage Labor to Women During Childbirth." It was written by Kathleen Rice Simpson, PhD, RNC, FAAN, for the *Journal of Perinatal Education.* You may be able to access it at *http://www.ncbi.nlm.nih.gov/pmc/articles/PMC1804305/* if the link is still current. Don't assume that your healthcare providers are aware of these guidelines—they may not be.

To sum this up, **here are some of the questions you'll want to ask your doctor or midwife:**

1. What position do you have women deliver their babies in? Also ask if they are open to other positions, like side-lying, modified squatting, standing, or on hands and knees.

2. How much time do you give a woman to deliver her baby before you encourage pushing? (Realize, however, that there are always medical considerations for the safety of the mother and child, so make it clear that you are aware of that, and that you agree that safety comes first.)

3. Do you encourage women to hold their breath when they are pushing? Or do you encourage them to push when they feel a contraction?

If you don't like your doctor's or midwife's answer, share with them the journal article I cited above. Chances are they'll welcome the new information and work with you to find the safest birthing positions and techniques for you.

Pack Your Hospital Bag for Comfort

Here are some terrific items to add to your hospital bag to ease pain and increase your comfort after you give birth. (We'll talk

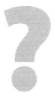

Did You Know…?

The best positions to deliver a baby are:
1. Side-Lying
2. Hands and Knees
3. Standing
4. Modified Squatting

about these more in an upcoming chapter on self-care immediately after giving birth.)

- ✦ At least two dozen **non-latex gloves.** (You'll pack these with ice and use them for pain relief, as I'll explain in Chapters Eight and Nine.)
- ✦ **Microwavable Moist Heating Pads. This will be handy to relieve neck and lower back pain** in the hospital and at home. Most hospitals will have a microwave you can use to heat them up.
- ✦ Special supportive garments that can help support your body after birth, such as the **Baby Bod® Abdominal Wrap, compression shorts** and a **Pelvic Floor Support Belt.** We will discuss these items in more detail in Chapter Eight and in Chapter Nine.
- ✦ A **small (12-inch by 12-inch) pillow**—pack one if you're having a *planned* Cesarean birth. You'll find it helpful to hold this pillow against your tummy when you cough, roll over in bed, or get out of bed.
- ✦ **Two tennis balls inside a tube sock** to be used to roll over sore muscles.
- ✦ A **donut-shaped pillow** to sit on. Find out if you will be provided one during your stay. If not, bring one with you and use it to decrease pain in your bottom caused by a vaginal delivery or hemorrhoids.
- ✦ Two extra pairs of **comfy socks**, a **zippered sweatshirt**, two or three **cotton nightgowns** that are designed to have easy access to your breasts for nursing, and a **robe** and **slippers.**
- ✦ Your **favorite pillow from home.** I found hospital pillows very uncomfortable after my first delivery and I was able to rest better when I brought my own pillow when I delivered my second child.

PLAN AHEAD

Arrange Now For Household Help after the Birth

Right now, you probably aren't thinking much at all about the condition your body will be in after you give birth. But I am—which is why I am urging you to talk with the baby's dad, your mom, sister and/or mother-in-law about arranging their schedule so they can give you some extra help with household chores once the baby comes. If you are lucky, you may be able to hire someone to help you. Ideally, you'll need extra help for at least the first six weeks. During that time, your soft tissue will still be healing. Your body will also be less stable than it was before, due to changes that occurred during pregnancy and delivery. You will also face the possibility of muscle and joint strain from repeated bending over to pick up your infant or hunching over to change diapers.[C]

While your body is still recovering, you'll need help with any household chores that require you to lift or push anything heavier than your baby. I'm talking about major grocery shopping, lifting a heavy laundry basket, taking a big pot off the stove, pushing a heavy vacuum cleaner, etc.

The rule of thumb—for at least the first six weeks after you deliver—is to avoid lifting or pushing anything heavier than your baby. It's a good idea to commit this guidance to memory now.

Plan ahead and ask now so you never find yourself in a position where you have no choice but to do a task that could potentially injure you.

Teach Any Older Children to Meet You "Half-Way"

If you already have young children at home, begin now to "train" them to climb up on the couch or a "cuddle chair" if they want a hug from you, or you need to dress them, or you want to pick them up. Make it a game: Tell them, "I'll race you to the cuddle chair." This way, after you have your new baby, you won't have to bend down so far to pick your toddler up. That will help spare your back and keep you from straining your abdominal and pelvic floor muscles. This is great if you're a working mom and you've gotten into the habit of picking up your child and hugging them when you arrive home from work. Get them to meet you at the cuddle chair instead.

The Rule of Thumb

Do not lift or push anything heavier than your newborn baby for the first 6 weeks after you had your baby.

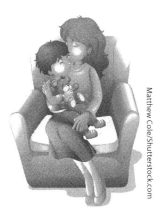

Matthew Cole/Shutterstock.com

[C] You'll really do your back a favor if you set up an "ergonomic" (body-friendly) nursery. Buying the right baby gear is important, but you also need to make sure you are using these items correctly to help prevent aches and pains. I cover this in depth in Chapters 16 and 17.

Consider Consulting a Physical Therapist Prior to Delivery

Most people don't realize that a physical therapist can help get your body ready for the rigors of childbirth. During your **birthing prep consultation**, your physical therapist will evaluate your body to see if there are some biomechanical problems that need to be addressed to make childbirth easier. More specifically, he or she can:

+ Help *relieve most of the aches and pains* you might be experiencing.
+ Give you one-on-one *advice on how to use your body* without causing strain on your back now and after you deliver your baby.
+ Evaluate your condition and develop a *specific exercise program* to prepare you for childbirth. (You can bring this book and ask your physical therapist to make sure that you are doing the **Baby Bod® exercises** correctly.)
+ Use *manual physical therapy* to ensure you are in the best condition possible when it comes time to deliver your child. This can make delivering your baby that much more comfortable for you, and easier on your body and baby, too.
+ Teach you *specific exercises to use while you are in labor* to ensure better alignment of the pelvis to help make birthing easier.[D]

A physical therapist or physiotherapist who has advanced training in treating the pelvic floor can also help you **determine what birthing position is best for you**. The therapist will place biofeedback sensors on your pelvic floor and have you move into several different positions while checking the results on a biofeedback machine. This will help determine the positions in which your pelvic floor muscles are most relaxed. Finding the birthing position that works best for you should help make your childbirth experience a lot more efficient and pleasant. For more information on how to find a physical therapist, see Appendix C in the back of the book.

* * *

[D] As part of birthing preparation, I like to teach my clients how to use "self-mobilization" techniques to perform at the start of labor and in between contractions to ensure better pelvic alignment. This seems to put the pelvis into the best position possible when it comes time to push the baby out.

I hope I've convinced you to read this book now, rather than set it aside until after you have your baby. You can start the **Baby Bod® Exercise Program** NOW to help prepare your body for the rigors of childbirth and to make it easier to resume it after you deliver your baby.

My very best wishes to you for a safe, happy, and healthy delivery!

[1] Labonte-Lemoynee E, Curnier D, Ellemberg D. Foetal brain development is influenced by maternal exercise during pregnancy. Paper presented at Kinesiology, Univ. of Montreal; November 10, 2013; Montreal, QC, Canada.

[2] Miquelutti MA, Cecatti JG, Makuch MY. Evaluation of a birth preparation program on lumbopelvic pain, urinary incontinence, anxiety and exercise: a randomized controlled trial. *BMC Pregnancy and Childbirth.* 2013; 13:154. http://www.biomedcentral.com/1471-2393/13/154

[3] Reynolds G. Mother's Exercise May Boost Baby's Brain. *New York Times.* November 20, 2013. http://well.blogs.nytimes.com/2013/11/20/mothers-exercise-may-boost-babys-brain/?_php=true&_type=blogs&_r=0

[4] Committee on Obstetric Practice. Exercise During Pregnancy and the Postpartum Period. *Obstet Gynecol.* 2009; 99: 171-173. http://www.acog.org/Resources_And_Publications/Committee_Opinions/Committee_on_Obstetric_Practice/Exercise_During_Pregnancy_and_the_Postpartum_Period

[5] Ryan M. Reducing the Risk of Pelvic Organ Prolapse: Birthing Techniques for Less Strain on Pelvic Floor Muscles. *Association for Pelvic Organ Prolapse Support.* http://www.pelvicorganprolapsesupport.org/birthing-techniques-for-less-strain-on-pelvic-floor-muscles/

[6] Simpson KR. When and How to Push: Providing the Most Current Information About Second-Stage Labor to Women During Childbirth Education. *J Perinat Educ.* 2006 Fall; 15(4): 6–9. doi: 10.1624/105812406X151367

Baby Bod® for New Moms: Help! I Just Got Home and Looked in the Mirror!

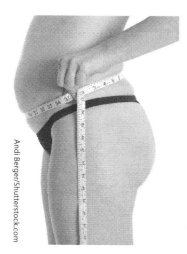

Andi Berger/Shutterstock.com

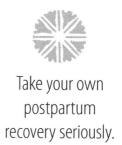

Take your own postpartum recovery seriously.

After the excitement of childbirth, first-time moms are often shocked to discover that their bodies don't automatically snap back into shape. The first thing I remember after I got home with my new baby was looking sideways in a mirror and gasping…I still looked pregnant! Was I ever going to see a flat tummy again!?! Wow, how unfair! How come I saw celebrities looking like hot babes shortly after they give birth?

First of all, expecting yourself to be "red-carpet ready" soon after delivering your baby is unrealistic for the normal everyday gal. It's not even normal for celebrities.

It will take time for your belly to shrink no matter who you are. So don't put yourself under the pressure to be "Facebook ready" two days after you deliver your baby!

Why does it seem celebrity moms look better faster? It's true that most can afford a lot of extra help, but more importantly, *they take postpartum recovery seriously.* You may not be able to afford a full-time nanny, night-time baby nurse, personal trainer, and a cook, but you too can take your own recovery seriously. So put aside all your pregnancy books and let your own postpartum needs come front and center. That's what Baby Bod® is for. It's time for YOU to get your pre-baby body back!

ABOUT THAT BOWLING BALL IN YOUR TUMMY POST-DELIVERY

Did you happen to see the video that captured the first appearance of Prince William and his wife, Catherine, the Duchess of Cambridge, when they presented their newborn baby, Prince George, to the world? It had only been one day since Kate had given birth and there was a huge crowd of people anxiously waiting to capture the first glimpse of the new heir to the throne. What a picture of a fairytale come true.

NOT!

As Kate lovingly passed her newborn son to Prince William, we all saw that her belly looked as if she were still six months pregnant. It was clear as day!

What's up with that?

This came as a surprise to the general public: Why did she still look pregnant after giving birth? Was there something wrong with the normally picture-perfect Kate? There was a media explosion after that and lots of discussions about the size of Kate's postpartum belly. People were surprised to learn that she looked perfectly normal for a woman who had just given birth.

The size of Kate's belly didn't come as a surprise to me. Few people realize that it's *normal* to still look pregnant for a few weeks or more after giving birth; I refer to this as the **Post-Baby Bowling-Ball Belly.** There are many internal and external changes in a woman's body after delivery. During pregnancy, normal women gain 40 to 50 percent more blood volume. All that excess fluid doesn't go away in a few hours. It can take at least a couple of weeks for the fluids you normally retain during pregnancy to reach a new balance in your body. That is one reason why I think it is so helpful for women to wear medical-grade, light compression undergarments right after childbirth, which help the body rid itself of fluids more quickly. We'll talk about these garments in depth in the self-care chapters.

And that's not all. Your uterus, which stretched to accommodate your growing baby, now has to shrink back down to its original size. That will happen gradually over time, and sometimes occurs more quickly if you breastfeed. Muscles that stretched during pregnancy also have to shrink back down. And the internal organs, such as the stomach, intestines and even the liver, which moved to accommodate the growing child, now have to move back into place. The skin, which stretched as your belly expanded, also has to tighten.

So…realistically…it takes at least a month for your body to start to get itself back together, usually longer for most women.

I thought Ceridwen Morris made an excellent point on Babble. com when she said: "Seeing Kate's big belly is an important reminder that the process of making and giving birth to a baby does not end at birth. The slow shifting, shrinking and drifting of various tissues and parts is appropriately gentle and very well designed. Of course it takes time!"[A]

Yes . . . it . . . does . . . But with the right holistic program you can help Nature along—that's the point of **Baby Bod®**. It will give you the results you want because it is grounded in an accurate understanding of what's amiss in the postpartum body and because it applies the best evidence-based solutions in a holistic way.

STEER CLEAR OF THE SCALE!

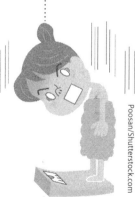

Whatever you do, don't even think of stepping on that scale for at least thirty days after you deliver your baby. I remember breaking down into tears after I weighed myself three days after I delivered my first daughter. I only lost a few pounds! How can that be? She weighed 8 ½ pounds and the placenta and amniotic fluid weighed about 3 or 4 pounds, so I should be at least 12 pounds less, right?

Wrong!

Here is why: Right after giving birth, your body is still going through hormonal changes. The amount of fluid your body retains can fluctuate hourly, especially if you are nursing. It takes a few weeks for your body to lose the excess fluid you build up during your pregnancy and for your uterus to return to normal size. So, as much fun as it may seem to find out how much you weigh, don't do it; it can drive you crazy.

Poosan/Shutterstock.com

[A] This quote is reprinted here with permission from Ceridwen Morris.

Baby Bod® applies the best evidence-based solutions for postpartum recovery in a holistic way.

If you're a new mom, you can skip the next chapter for experienced moms and go straight to Chapter Four on anatomy, and start to learn a little bit about your postpartum body. Also, be sure to read the three chapters that follow rather than skipping right to the self-care or exercise chapters. These chapters are MUST READS for you. They'll help you better understand what is different in your body now as a woman who has undergone nine months of progressive physical change during pregnancy and the birth experience. They'll also give you a handle on any post-birth problems you may be experiencing now or could well experience down the road if you don't take the appropriate steps to stop any developing disorder. The better informed you are, the less likely you are to fall prey to bad advice that could set your recovery back, such as that from well-meaning fitness or even healthcare professionals who urge you to do sit-ups, or the celebrity moms who enthusiastically endorse abdominal binders. Neither of these is good for postpartum women, for reasons I will explain as we go along.

The better informed you are, the less likely you are to fall prey to bad advice that could set your recovery back.

CHAPTER THREE

Baby Bod® for Experienced Moms: "Once Postpartum, Always Postpartum"®

The stresses and strains of pregnancy and childbirth do more than create that "Mommy Tummy;" they can also lead to pain in the back, pelvis and, yes, a leaky bladder. Not all of these changes show up right after you deliver your baby. Studies show that it can take years for some of these symptoms to develop into problems.[1] This can happen even if you feel great after you have your baby.

So ladies, while it may come as a shock to hear this, you may not feel these effects until after your child enrolls in kindergarten or graduates from college.

That's not good news, I know, but I'm about to tell you something that may make you feel better. **Baby Bod®** can help you fully recover, even if it's been years since you gave birth. It will address *hidden internal problems* that began when you were pregnant or right after birth, and that have been silently and slowly getting worse ever since. It can also prevent them from becoming full-blown medical disorders.

Consider this: Once you have a baby, you are always "postpartum." As I always tell my clients, ***"Once Postpartum, Always Postpartum."®*** And it's never too late to get your postpartum body back in shape.

* * *

Every day in my practice, I see women who have developed incontinence or pain in their backs and pelvises, and they are absolutely shocked when I tell them that it is all a result of childbirth years or even decades earlier.

It's never too late to get your postpartum body back in shape.

My client, Alice, is typical. She had terrible pelvic pain for several years and saw many doctors before one finally diagnosed the cause of the pain: *pelvic scar tissue*. This was related to a traumatic birth injury forty-two years before. Her gynecologist referred her to me, and I did manual therapy (hands-on work) to control the pain. Then I recommended five strategies, including the exercises in the **Baby Bod® Program**, that she could use to help diminish the pain and restore her ability to function on the job and daily commute. She faithfully followed my advice, and is now pain free and extremely grateful. (She tells me I have "magic hands!")

As you can see, with a little help from physical therapy and some daily homework, Alice was able to recover from the damage that was done over four decades earlier when she had a very difficult delivery with severe vaginal tears. Even though she was not in pain until years later, the damage she sustained to the support system that holds up her internal organs just kept getting progressively worse—similar to the way a small tear in a pair of stockings eventually becomes a gaping hole—until things deteriorated to the point where it caused her real problems. I've shared her story because I want to give every reader who is in pain hope again. This program and physical therapy, if necessary—and it often is—can help resolve pain that developed as a result of childbirth, even if you gave birth decades ago!

With the right help, it's never too late to fully recover from pregnancy and labor. I am a prime example. It took me a few decades to figure out how to resolve my incontinence and pelvic pain, but once I had the solution, both were gone for good.

Baby Bod® Can Prevent Menopause-Related Prolapse

This program—again, perhaps in conjunction with physical therapy if needed—can also save you older moms from another headache—pelvic organ prolapse (POP).[2, 3] A study[4] involving older women with an average age of fifty-three years (about half of the women in this group were menopausal) found that one half of them had pelvic organ prolapse. The women who had POP also had a higher incidence of pelvic floor dysfunctions such as pelvic pain and incontinence (urine and fecal leakage).

***

Pelvic Organ Prolapse – Menopause

Pelvic Organ Prolapse can happen during menopause, too. As estrogen levels decline, the tissue becomes less elastic. As the ligaments lose their elasticity, they become stretched out and provide less support, which leads to a downward migration of the pelvic organs. So if you have an older friend or grandmother, you might mention that **Baby Bod®** can help her too. If that doesn't do the trick, she might want to consult a pelvic physical therapist.

***

Childbirth isn't the only instigator; pelvic organ prolapse can also develop as one of the negative side effects of menopause.[5] Studies have shown the right pelvic floor exercises can reverse prolapse, or at the very least, improve the condition.[2, 3] If that has occurred to you, try Baby Bod® first. If that doesn't do the trick, consult a pelvic physical therapist or woman's health physiotherapist.

That's your best bet. Why does it work?[2] Well, the deep, core muscles in your body connect to the deep ligaments that suspend your internal organs, especially the bladder, uterus and rectum. So if you learn how to do the correct exercises, which strengthen the muscles that support your pelvic organs, you can tighten up the entire suspension system that begins to slip downwards during menopause.

This is a much better course of action than surgery for pelvic organ prolapse, which has a high failure rate. A recent study (2013) funded by the National Health Institutes showed that nearly one-third of women who underwent an operation called a *sacrocolpopex* to correct pelvic organ prolapse and incontinence found that the problems the surgery was supposed to fix permanently came back within just SEVEN years.[6] (THAT IS NOT A GOOD STATISTIC!)

I'll talk about POP in more in depth in Chapter Seven. Before I leave this subject, however, I want to make sure that you know—especially if you are planning to have another child or know someone who is pregnant and can use this information—that the best way to prevent POP is by using the best possible birthing techniques. This way, there's less likelihood that the vaginal walls or pelvic muscles are torn. That's what sets the stage for later trouble. (For more information on this, see "The Right Birthing Techniques Now Can Spare You Misery Later" in Chapter One.)

Here's more good news for you older moms: If you are starting the program months, years, or even decades after you had your last baby, you can get through it faster than women who have just given birth. I want you to learn all the **Preliminary Phase Exercises** (you'll find these in Chapters Eleven to Fourteen) and then perform them for one solid week consistently. After that, you can go onto the **Advanced Phase – Strengthening Exercises** in Chapter Fifteen.

Before you go to the exercise chapters, however, please do read the next few chapters, which will explain what has happened to your lady parts and belly. Don't skip them! This information and the accompanying illustrations will help you understand the exercise directions better so you can do the exercises correctly. I also want you to do the self-massages in Chapter Eight if you had a vaginal delivery, or Chapter Nine if you had a C-section. They'll help you, no matter how long it's been since you've had your baby.

With the right help, it's never too late to fully recover from pregnancy and delivery.

[1] Sapsford R. Rehabilitation of pelvic floor muscles utilizing trunk stabilization. *Manual Therapy.* 2004 Feb; 9(1):3-12.

[2] Hagen S, Stark D. Conservative prevention and management of pelvic organ prolapse in women. *Cochrane Database Syst Rev.* 2011 Dec 7; (12):CD003882. doi: 10.1002/14651858.CD003882.pub4.

[3] Braekken IH, Majida M, Ellström EM, Holme IM, Bo K. Pelvic floor function is independently associated with pelvic organ prolapse. *BJOG.* 2009 Dec; 116(13):1706-14. doi: 10.1111/j.1471-0528.2009.02379.x.

[4] Spitnagle TM, Leong FC, Van Dillen LR. Prevalence of diastasis rectus abdominis in a urogynecological patient population. *Int Urogynecol J.* 2007 ; 18(3):321-8. doi:10.1007/s00192-006-0143-5

[5] Dietz HP. Prolapse worsens with age, doesn't it? *Aust. N. Z. J. Obstet. Gynaecol.*2008; 48(6): 587–591. doi: 10.1111/j.1479-828X.2008.00904.x.

[6] Nygaard I, Brubaker L, Zyczynski HM, et al. Long-term outcomes following abdominal sacrocolpopexy for pelvic organ prolapse. JAMA. 2013 May 15; 309(19):2016-24. doi: 10.1001/*JAMA*.2013.4919.

About that Anatomy Lesson…

Even if you have read TONS about the changes that occur during pregnancy and delivery, I'd bet that no one has satisfactorily explained to you how all these changes affect your body *after* you have given birth. I will share that knowledge with you over the next several chapters. You're going to need it to understand how to flatten that tummy in the shortest time possible.

In this chapter, I want to go over some basic anatomy with you. This will serve a double purpose. First, it will give you a context for understanding what has changed. Second, it will help you identify some of the less familiar parts of the body that you will need to locate to do the **Baby Bod® exercises** correctly.

We'll start by going over the bony structures most affected by pregnancy—the pelvis, ribcage, and spine—and then proceed to the muscles. (Don't skip over this; you'll need to know every bit of this to do the exercises correctly.) To make it easier on you to learn this mini- anatomy lesson, I've included illustrations throughout. If you forget where a body part is located when you are reading the exercise instructions, you can always flip back to this chapter.

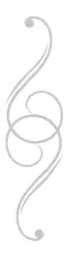

Don't skip over this; you'll need to know every bit of this to do the exercises correctly.

THE PELVIC GIRDLE

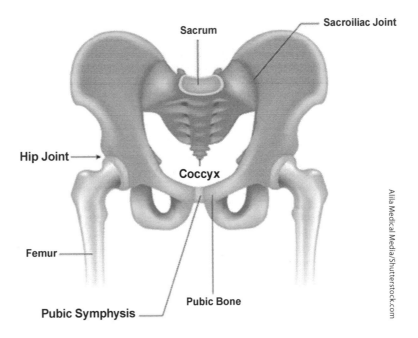

Sacrum

Sacroiliac Joint

Hip Joint

Coccyx

Femur

Pubic Bone

Pubic Symphysis

Alila Medical Media/Shutterstock.com

LOCATING THE PELVIS, SPINE, AND RIBCAGE

Pelvis

As you can see in the illustration, the pelvis is mainly made up of three large bony parts. Two of the bones are U-shaped; they wrap around the sides of your torso and meet in the front to form a joint called the *pubic symphysis*. (I will refer to this part of the pelvis in some of the exercises, so please make a mental note of where your pubic symphysis is located. On occasion, I will also refer to the pubic symphysis area as your *pubic bone*.)

The *pubic symphysis joint* is made up of a large piece of cartilage, which serves to separate the front of the pelvis into right and left sides. Since cartilage is softer then bone, this arrangement helps to make the front of the pelvis flexible. The hormones produced during pregnancy make the pubic symphysis even more flexible, which means it can move more than it did before you conceived. If the joint moves too much, which is more likely to happen toward the last trimester of pregnancy, it can cause pain. (This is referred to as **Pubic Symphysis Dysfunction**.) Postpartum women can also develop pain in this area, especially after a vaginal delivery. (I will talk more about this—and what you can do for this kind of pain—in Chapter Six.)

On the sides, the two U-shaped bones form the sockets of the *hip joints*. This is where the legs attach to the pelvis.

The U-shaped bones also curve around to the back of the body where they each connect to a triangular-shaped bone called the *sacrum*. The *sacroiliac joints* are formed at this connection. At the bottom of the sacrum is the *coccyx*, or tailbone. Many postpartum clients of mine have told me they experienced pain in the coccyx while they were pregnant and after childbirth. If the coccyx it twisted, bruised or broken during childbirth, it can be painful to sit.

The sacrum is the anatomical structure the *lumbar spine* rises up from. The spine is made up of many small bones called *vertebra*, which stack up one on top of the other. There are five *lumbar vertebrae*, which form the area that is typically referred to as the lower back. Above that is the *thoracic spine*, which is made up of twelve vertebrae that attach to the *rib cage*. Above the ribcage are seven *cervical vertebrae* that form the neck.

SPINE, RIB CAGE AND PELVIS

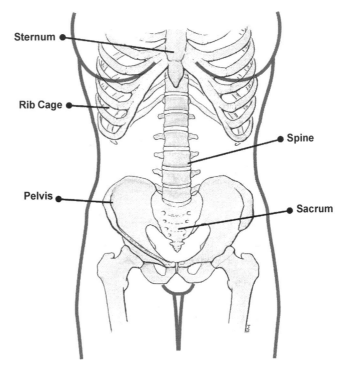

Sternum

Rib Cage

Spine

Pelvis

Sacrum

Spine and Rib Cage

The *ribcage* is made up of twelve ribs; it attaches to your spine in the back. The breastbone or *sternum* is on the front part of the ribcage (as shown in the illustration below).

I'd like you to take a moment to look at the illustration above and locate the bottom of the sternum in the front of your ribcage on your own body. (Note the placement of the uppermost hand in the picture.) The sternum is in the middle of the front of your rib cage, where the softer part of your abdomen meets a harder area, the bottom of your rib cage.

Next, locate your pubic symphysis or "pubic bone." That's the hard area just below your panty line. When I teach you a few of the exercises, I'll ask you to place your hands on your sternum and pubic bone, so please make a mental note of where they are.

In a well-functioning body, the pelvis, spine and rib cage are in the correct alignment to each other when you move and when you are at rest. In an upcoming chapter, I will teach you how to get your alignment right, a practice that automatically gets your core muscles to work optimally with little effort on your part.

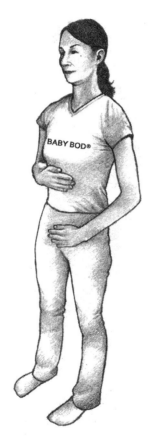

Locate your *pubic symphysis* (pubic bone) and *sternum*

I will teach you how to get your alignment right, a practice that automatically gets your core muscles to work optimally with little effort on your part.

Learning More About the Pelvic Floor

I would also like you to familiarize yourself with the *pelvic floor*. You'll need to know this later when I teach you how to feel for a muscular contraction at the bottom of your pelvis. You will also need to do this in one of the first exercises you will learn in the **Preliminary Phase of Baby Bod®**. When we get there, if you're not sure where to place your hand, you can refer back to this illustration.

The *pelvic floor* is made up of soft tissue and muscle. It's called the "floor" because it is at the bottom of the pelvis. It lies in between your pubic symphysis (in the front of the pelvis) and your coccyx (your tail bone, in the back). As you'll see in the illustration below, in women, the pelvic floor is diamond-shaped. The outer layer is made up of soft tissue, which is split down the middle and forms the *labia*. The *pelvic floor muscles* lie underneath this soft tissue. The *anus, vagina* and *urethra* protrude through openings in the pelvic floor

If you look closely at the picture below, the *perineum* is the soft tissue that separates and lies in-between the vagina and the anus. This is one of the most common areas that can tear during childbirth. This is also the area that is cut when the obstetrician performs an episiotomy during delivery.

OUTER PELVIC FLOOR

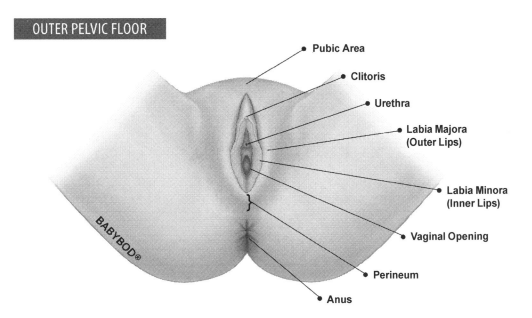

PELVIC FLOOR MUSCLES

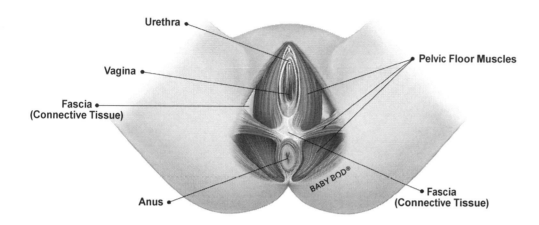

THE MUSCLES

Now that you're acquainted with the important skeletal structures, let's look more closely at the muscles that are most affected by pregnancy and childbirth. These are the muscles that you will target in the **Baby Bod® Program**: the muscles that you need to work on to flatten your tummy.

Pelvic Floor Muscles

These muscles lie at the bottom of your pelvis. They are made up of several intertwining muscle fibers that almost form a figure eight around your genitals and rectum. (See illustration above.) These muscles—along with the *fascia* that make up the pelvic floor—support the bladder, uterus, and rectum. The openings for the urethra, the vagina and the anus pass through these interwoven muscles. When pelvic floor muscles are strong and functioning optimally, they help you control bladder and bowel function. They also play an important role in sexual function.

One thing I would like you to note here is that there is a lot of fascia interwoven in the pelvic floor muscles. The fascia is made up of sheets of supportive connective tissue and resembles the white tissue you can easily see in pieces of red meat. The fascia in the pelvic floor separates and supports the pelvic organs, such as the uterus, bladder and rectum. It plays a major role in supporting the bottom of the pelvis, and helps to hold the muscles in place so they don't droop downwards like "droopy drawers."

Did You Know?

Normally, most people think of a muscle as one solid mass of tissue, kind of like what you see at the butcher shop when the butcher is cutting up a side of beef or leg of lamb. But what you see in the butcher shop is several different muscles grouped together and wrapped around a bone. An individual muscle is actually made up of layer upon layer of muscular fibers, and each muscle is held together in a "bunch" by connective tissue. Then there are layers of fascia, which is made up of connective tissue, that serve to separate and support the muscles. The body has so much muscle tissue, in fact, that muscle tissue normally accounts for about 40-45 percent of our body weight.

THE ABDOMINAL MUSCLES: "THERE IS MORE THAN MEETS THE EYE"

Two Layers of Abdominal Muscles:

As you can see in the illustration further down in this section, your tummy is made up of several layers of muscles. To simplify things, I like to explain that there are two distinctive layers of abdominal muscles: an outer layer and inner layer of muscles. These two layers of abdominal muscles function differently. The *outer muscles* function as "**movers**" while the *inner layer of muscle* "**holds**" things together. The deepest layer of abdominal muscles, the *transverse abdominis,* is part of the core muscle system and one of its main functions is to hold your internal organs in place. We will get into more detail about core muscles later on in the book.

To understand the difference between the **outer muscles** and the **inner muscles** in the abdomen, it might help to look closely at the illustration further down in this section. The cutaway in the illustration will help you see the different layers of muscles. You can easily see that the abdomen is made up of four layers of muscles. The three layers that are closest to the surface are the *outer abdominal muscles* and the deepest layer is the *inner abdominal muscle.*

It's important to understand the distinction between the inner and outer muscles; ultimately, you need to do slightly different things to each to restore them after the rigors of pregnancy and childbirth. Let's look more closely at each layer further down in this section.

The outer muscles function as "movers" while the inner layer of muscle "holds" things together.

LAYERS OF ABDOMINAL MUSCLES

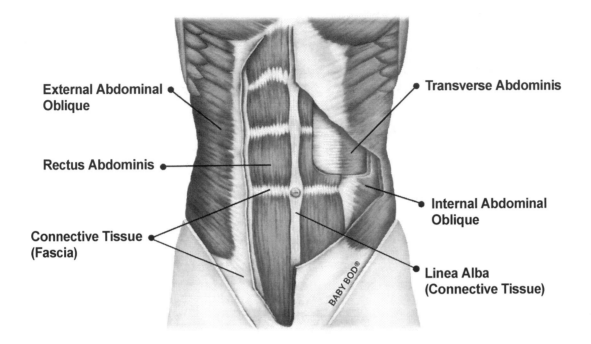

External Abdominal Oblique

Rectus Abdominis

Connective Tissue (Fascia)

Transverse Abdominis

Internal Abdominal Oblique

Linea Alba (Connective Tissue)

BABY BOD®

The Outer Layer of Abdominal Muscles

There are three muscles that form the outer layer of abdominal muscles; they work together to bend or curl your chest towards your pelvis and to rotate your torso:

1. *External Abdominal Obliques*: These lie on both sides of your abdomen. They are often called the "love handle" muscles.

2. *Internal Abdominal Obliques*: Beneath the external oblique is a layer of muscle called the *internal abdominal oblique*.

3. *Rectus Abdominis*: In the very front of the abdomen, you'll find the *rectus abdominis*, the so-called "six-pack" muscle, which looks almost like two large ribbons running down the front of the

abdomen on either side of the belly button. The rectus abdominis muscle is separated by connective tissue, which is called the *linea alba*. (You can see the linea alba in the illustration above; it's the thin white band running right down the center of the abdomen.) During pregnancy, this connective tissue, which is looser than it was before you became pregnant, often expands and spreads apart to accommodate the size of the growing baby. As the linea alba expands, the two rectus abdominis muscles slide further apart. If the stretching out of the linea alba causes too much of a gap between these muscles, it creates a condition known as *diastasis recti*. (*Diastasis* comes from a Latin word that means the abnormal separation of parts normally joined together.) I will talk much more about diastasis recti in Chapter Seven and tell you what you can do about it.

The Inner Layer of Abdominal Muscle – The Transverse Abdominis

Glance again at the illustration above and note that the deepest layer of muscle in the abdomen is called the **transverse abdominis**. As you can see in the illustration below, it wraps around the torso from front to back and from the ribs to the pelvis, forming a deep *corset of support*. Even though this muscle lies deep in the abdomen, it plays an important role in flattening your tummy.

When the transverse abdominis is working properly, it helps to stabilize (or "hold together") the pelvis and spine as you move. It also compresses the internal organs and helps to hold them in place. When it's working optimally, it creates a "scooping effect" in your lower abdomen, making your waist and tummy look tighter and flatter. Training this muscle—the correct way—will also help you get rid of that bulge in the bottom of your tummy. In the **Baby Bod® Exercise Program**, you will learn very specific exercises that target the transverse abdominis so that you can regain your pre-pregnancy waistline.

TRANSVERSE ABDOMINIS MUSCLE

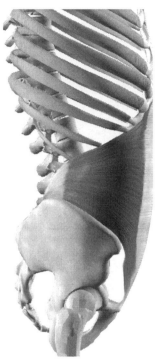

The transverse abdominis muscle does not work on its own to flatten your tummy. As I mentioned earlier, it belongs to a group of muscles referred to as the "*core muscles,*" a term you have probably heard. Also included in the core muscle group are the **pelvic floor muscles**; and two other muscles I will describe below; the *multifidus muscles*, the deepest layer of back muscles; and the *diaphragm*, the breathing muscle that separates the abdomen from the chest.

These muscles are called "core" because they are the deepest muscles in your body and lie in the core of your body. They are considered a group because they work together in coordinated fashion rather than independently. One of the main functions of the core muscles is to hold your torso together as you move around. I will discuss how the core muscles function in more detail in Chapter Six.

Let's take a brief look at the two core muscles I haven't yet described.

Multifidus Muscles – The Deepest Layer of Back Muscles

As you can see in the illustration below, the *multifidus muscles* travel the entire length of the spine; they start at the sacrum (in the back of the pelvis) and continue upwards to the back of your skull. Notice that they extend, in the mid-back area, to the sides of the rib cage. These are the deepest layer of back muscles and they serve to stiffen or "hold" the spine together during virtually all movements. If your multifidus muscles were not working properly, the spine would move too much each time you bent down to pick up a piece of paper or turned to look at something interesting in a store window. You wouldn't feel stable. When this group of muscles is working properly, however, it holds your spine together so that you can move your entire body as one unit.

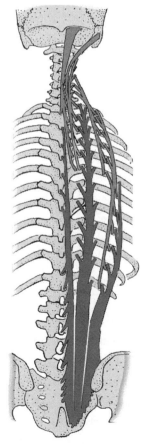

MULTIFIDUS MUSCLE

The multifidus muscles run up both sides of your spine, the illustration only shows the multifidus on the right side of the body.

`DIAPHRAGM`

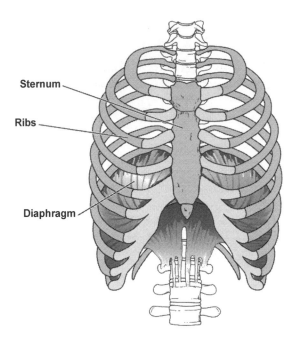

Sternum

Ribs

Diaphragm

Blamb/Shutterstock.com

The Diaphragm

This large, dome-shaped muscle separates your stomach and other internal organs from the lungs. You may think of it as a breathing muscle only—and that *is* its main function (driving the mechanics of breathing)—but most people are surprised to learn that it also serves as a core muscle. The way you breathe causes the pressure in your belly to change automatically as you go about your daily activities. This is when the diaphragm has the most influence over the other core muscles. (I will discuss this in more detail in Chapter Six.) Since you want the pressure to be just right, your diaphragm has to work as efficiently as possible.

During the latter stages of pregnancy, the growing uterus pushes up against the diaphragm, preventing the diaphragm from working to full capacity. The baby gains more room, but your breathing becomes shallower and less efficient as a result. And in the process, your diaphragm isn't able to contribute as a core muscle.

So after you give birth, you have to take the right steps to restore the diaphragm's ability to work at full capacity again. That's why it is *so* important to do breathing exercises—like the super-targeted ones I will teach you—after you have your baby. The **Baby Bod® Program** breathing exercises I will teach you in Chapter Twelve will help restore both the breathing and core supportive functions of the diaphragm.

* * *

That's it for the basic anatomy primer. You'll build upon this knowledge in the next two chapters, where we will look at hidden changes in the postpartum body that you need to address to accelerate your recovery.

CHAPTER FIVE

Why Your Body Doesn't Just "Snap Back" Afterwards

Oh that poor, *misunderstood*, misshapen postpartum belly. "Is this just fat?" you wonder when you catch a glimpse of your naked belly in the mirror. "When is it going to look normal again?"

Let me let you in on a little secret that few moms know: No, it is not "just fat." There are other factors that can make the postpartum belly bulge and/or sag, and that's what we're going to talk about in this chapter. You need to know what they are so that you can intelligently and actively support your body as it heals. By the time you finish this chapter, I promise you, you'll understand exactly why your body doesn't just "snap back" to its pre-pregnancy condition and what steps you can take to ensure a fabulous recovery!

Older moms, please read this chapter, too. It's possible that your body has never fully recovered from pregnancy and birth—something I see again and again in my practice. Some moms, for instance, still have that "Mommy Tummy" many years after they gave birth to their last child. Do you? If so, the two self-tests I provide below will give you some very useful information about where your recovery may have stalled.

THE POST-BABY BOWLING-BALL-BELLY PHASE

One of the factors that makes the belly bulge out is fluid retention, and it affects moms in the immediate aftermath of birth. As I said earlier in the book, it can take a month or so for your uterus and muscles to shrink back down and to lose the extra fluids you retained during pregnancy. (As I said in the chapter for new moms, one of the best ways to get the body to shed that fluid faster is to make smart use of graduated compression garments, something I will

Intelligently and actively support your body as it heals and recovers from pregnancy.

talk about at length in Chapters Eight and Nine.)

Once you get through that early "post-baby bowling-ball-belly phase" and your tummy is no longer swollen, you're still not out of the woods, however. At that point, you may still have a sagging belly and what feels like several pounds of soft, gelatinous blubber forming an undesirable bulge in your lower abdomen.

YOUR STABILITY SYSTEM – YOUR "CORE"[A]

What causes the belly to sag and/or the lower abdomen to bulge out *after* the body rids itself of excess fluid? The answer to this is a little more complicated, but it has to do with the current state of your abdominal muscles and connective tissue, and the influence of hormones on that tissue. I will explain this bit by bit. Stay with me. What I am about to tell you may be the most critical piece of information missing from your understanding of your postpartum body.

Your muscles and connective tissue are part of a larger system in the body, the *"Stability System."*[1, 2] This is the system that keeps you upright and prevents your internal organs from falling out of your "lady parts" after birth whenever you stand up.

Unfortunately, it can become compromised during pregnancy, childbirth, and beyond. If this system is compromised and your abdominal muscles are not working up to par, you probably won't be thrilled with how your belly looks.

The stability system is made up of three parts.[1, 3, 4] To make this even clearer, you are able to remain upright and move without falling apart at the seams because of:

1. The way your *bones* are shaped and the way they interlock. (Think of interlocking Lego blocks that snap together.) This provides the first level of stability.

[A] Special thanks to two physiotherapists for helping me figure out how to explain the stability system in simpler terms: Anthony Lo, The Phyiso Detective, APA Muscloskeletal Physiotherapist (www.physiodetective.com) and Diane Lee, BSR FCAMT RY200 (www.dianelee.ca).

2. The *connective tissue*, which includes ligaments, tendons, cartilage and that white fibrous stuff, called fascia, that you see when you cut up red meat. Connective tissue connects bone-to-bone (forming joints), supports muscles, and holds your organs in place. This forms the second level of stability.

3. The hundreds of *muscles* that wrap around the organs and bones provide the third level of stability. The muscles that offer you stability are the *core muscles*, the deeper network of muscles that I spoke about in the last chapter. Core muscles differ from the outer muscles in your body; their main function is to hold your body together and to keep you stable when you move around. (The outer muscles help you move.) If you want a flat belly, these muscles have to be functioning at 100 percent.

The *brain* controls the *synchronization* of all of these parts, working much like the folks at air traffic control in the airport, so its connection to all three of these is vitally important here. Each part of this three-level stability system relies on the others. If one part of this system is not working properly, the entire stability system fails and you lose the secure hold that is needed for smooth, efficient, and safe movement.

Ideally, your bones are in the correct alignment and fit snugly together, your ligaments and connective tissue are taut enough to hold your bones and muscles together, your organs are in place, and your muscles are just the right length and not stretched out. That enables the muscles to be strong when they contract.

Think of the stability system as a large jigsaw puzzle. In a well-functioning body, when you move, the stability system works to keep things in place so you can move around efficiently with the greatest amount of power.

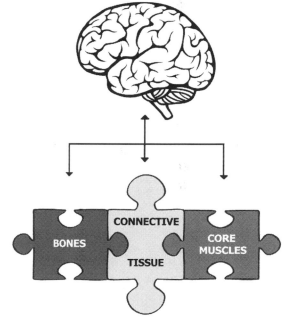

The brain controls and synchronizes the functioning of the stability system.

HOW PREGNANCY, BIRTH AND NURSING CAN TEMPORARILY MAKE THE BODY LESS STABLE AND MAKE YOUR TUMMY BULGE

As you know, during pregnancy, your body undergoes changes so that you can carry and deliver your child. Your entire abdomen —including your muscles and ligaments—becomes stretched out as your baby grows. The joints holding your pelvic bones together become a bit wobblier because the ligaments holding the pelvis together become looser. The connective tissue that supports your abdomen and muscles loosens up, which makes the muscles weaker.

"Pregnancy Hormones"

When you are pregnant, your body produces hormones that help the baby grow, help your body adapt to the ever-increasing size of the baby, and help prepare your body for childbirth[B]. Let's call them *"pregnancy hormones,"*[C] an idea I got after several email discussions with Dianne Edmonds, a well-respected Australian Women's Health Physiotherapist. (Thank you, Dianne!)

"Pregnancy hormones" work together to make the ligaments and the connective tissues that support the bones and muscles looser and more pliable so they can stretch out as the baby grows.[5,6] These hormones also allow the joints connecting the pelvic bones to loosen up to get your body ready for delivery. It is a gradual process, and as the baby grows, the joints connecting the pelvic bones become more flexible. By the time labor comes around, the pelvic bones spread as much as possible to widen the diameter of your pelvis so the baby can make its way down the birthing canal.

This is helpful when it comes time to push your baby through a

Most women do not realize their body is still under the influence of the "pregnancy hormones" for a good while after childbirth.

[B] There is a lot of controversy and many conflicting reports on which hormones cause ligaments and connective tissue to become looser during pregnancy and in postpartum women. Instead of identifying one hormone, I will be referring to them collectively as the "pregnancy hormones."

[C] Let me properly credit Dianne Edmonds for this term. She is the former National Chair of Continence and Women's Health Physiotherapy for the Australian Physiotherapy Association and was also a representative on the board of the International Organization of Physical Therapists in Women's Health [IOPTWH]. She was the Lead Physiotherapist and Special Projects Officer for the Pelvic Floor First Campaign for the Continence Foundation of Australia and is currently a campaign ambassador. Diane Edmond's website address is www.thepregnancycentre.com.au.

canal that normally stretches a few inches at most. That is one of the miracles of birth, isn't it?

The Lingering Effects of the "Pregnancy Hormones"

That's the upside. One of the downsides of these changes, however, is that it becomes harder for your body to maintain *stability*. The muscles and ligaments are stretched out and the joints holding the bones together are "wobblier," making you more prone to developing aches and pains during your pregnancy.

What most women do not realize is that their body is still under the influence of the "pregnancy hormones" for a good while *after* childbirth. It takes a while for the "pregnancy hormones" to dissipate, and that is one of the reasons why your body doesn't "snap back" to normal right after childbirth. *The joints, connective tissue and muscles can remain looser for some time after childbirth,* which means it can be harder to remain stable when you are a new mom. This is also the reason most women have bulging "Mommy Tummies" for a few months or more after childbirth. Obviously, if the connective tissue and muscle in your abdominal area remain loose, it will affect how your belly looks. It also means you are at increased risk of developing or aggravating one or more medical conditions—such as a leaky bladder, pelvic or back pain, or diastasis recti[D] (which is also sometimes called "Mommy Tummy").

How long are we talking about? The exact time a woman's body is under the influence of the "pregnancy hormones" depends on the individual[E] Some women may have systems that recover faster

---

[D] Diastasis recti is a condition where the abdominal muscles in the front of the abdomen spread apart, and cause the bulge many women develop in their bellies after childbirth, AKA the "Mommy Tummy." To read more about it, refer to Chapter 7.

[E] At time this book was published, there was very LIMITED research available about how long the connective tissue system remains compromised after childbirth. The best I can offer is to tell you what I have seen in my 30+ years of clinical experience working with pregnant and postpartum women. Typically, I have seen most women remain "looser" for a few months after they deliver their babies. If they are lactating mothers, they typically remain looser during the entire time they are nursing and for a few months after they wean their child. I have had several discussions with well-respected physical therapists and physiotherapists who reported seeing the same lingering effects of the "pregnancy hormones" on postnatal women, and we all agreed that more research is needed on the prolonged effects of the "pregnancy hormones" on postnatal women.

than others, while others take longer to recuperate. For example, women who have hypermobile body types (AKA: "double jointed") tend to remain looser longer. In general, however, if you are bottle-feeding, expect the "pregnancy hormones" to continue to exert their influence *for approximately three months after you give birth.* That means that you can remain "looser" and less stable for three months after you give birth. Breastfeeding mothers are under the influence of the "pregnancy hormones" for an even longer period of time than moms who bottle-feed their children. If you are nursing, *expect the lingering effects of the "pregnancy hormones" to last the entire time you are nursing and perhaps for as long as three months after you stop nursing.*

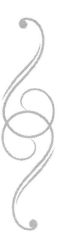

Eventually, that influence wears off and the joints, ligaments, and muscles firm up again. The tummy, however, does not always flatten automatically. But it will flatten if you take the correct steps, which **Baby Bod®** will walk you through. If you supply the effort, **Baby Bod®** can take you to full recovery.

THE LINGERING EFFECTS OF THE "PREGNANCY HORMONES"

Bottle Feeding Mothers	Breastfeeding Mothers
"Pregnancy hormones" can continue to affect connective tissue for up to 3 months after childbirth.	"Pregnancy hormones" can continue to affect connective tissue during the entire time you are nursing and for up to 3 months after you wean your child.
Stability system may be compromised for 3 months after childbirth.	Stability system may be compromised while lactating and for 3 months after you wean your child.
Take extra precautions during the first 3 months after childbirth to prevent injuries.	Take extra precautions to prevent injuries during the entire time you are nursing and for 3 months after you stop.

It's important to keep this in mind because a lot of moms wrongly assume that once they have their six-week postpartum check-up and hear their healthcare practitioner tell them that everything "looks fine," they can go back to "business as usual." **Not** true. In fact, six weeks allows for just the initial stage of recovery. That might be enough time for any soft tissue injuries to heal, but it's not enough time for the muscles to recover, and certainly not enough time for the connective tissue to completely firm up. As I just explained, that can take several months or more, depending upon whether or not you are breastfeeding. **Until the effects of the "pregnancy hormones" wear off, you need to avoid any activity that is too challenging for your current condition, or you could injure yourself.**

For instance, if you do something that places strain on your abdominal muscles before they have a chance to recover from childbirth, you could cause or aggravate diastasis recti, *which will make that "Mommy Tummy"* look even worse! Doing more than your body can handle—at the moment—can also cause you to develop or aggravate medical conditions such as incontinence, pelvic or back pain, or pelvic organ prolapse. [F, 7, 8, 9, 10] Why take the risk when a little understanding and patience can prevent all of this? (I'll go into detail about each of these conditions in Chapter Seven.)

The Dangers of Doing Too Much, Too Soon • A Case Story

Here's a cautionary tale that will make it very clear what could happen if you do too much, too soon. Megan was referred to me after her doctor diagnosed her with pelvic organ prolapse, which she developed *after* her six-week checkup.

Before she got pregnant, Megan was very active. She loved "boot camp-style" exercise programs and did half-marathons. After she got pregnant, severe nausea during her first trimester slowed her down some. To keep in shape, she started using the elliptical machine for cardio and doing lower-impact exercises such as yoga. Fortunately

Why take the
risk when a little
understanding
and patience can
prevent injuries?

[F] Pelvic organ prolapse is a condition where the pelvic organs, such as the uterus, bladder and bowels, slip down from their normal positions inside the pelvis and push down towards the pelvic floor. This condition can lead to developing incontinence and pelvic pain. Read more about it in Chapter 7.

for her, she had an easy vaginal delivery with just a few tears that needed stitching. She sailed right through her six-week postpartum checkup and was overjoyed when her doctor said she was fine and could return to all of her normal activities. Megan, being Megan, decided to start working out the next day.

Megan started with what she *thought* was an easy routine: running a few miles on the treadmill, working out with some weights, and doing crunches, Pilates-Hundred style. Right after her first workout, she felt something odd, as if she had a "golf ball" in her vagina. But she ignored it and kept up her daily workouts. Two weeks after she started working out, she went straight from the gym to the grocer and carried two heavy grocery bags up three flights of stairs to her apartment. When she got to the top of the stairs, she lost control of her bladder and wet herself. Worse yet, she felt a distinct bulge coming out of her vagina. When she checked herself with a mirror, Megan said she saw "part of her insides poking out of her vagina."

She got in to see the doctor immediately. The doctor told her she had pelvic organ prolapse; her bladder was falling into her vaginal canal and protruding out of it. Yikes! To treat her, the doctor put her on estrogen cream for several months. (Typically, estrogen helps keep the pelvic floor muscles toned, so they can support the pelvic organs. Because Megan was breastfeeding, her body was producing very little estrogen naturally.) The doctor also referred her to me for physical therapy.

See? This is what can happen if you go back to "business as usual" after your six week postpartum checkup and you ask your body to do more than it can presently handle.

Fortunately, Megan's story had a happy ending. I initially saw her for two and a half months.

I taught her how to do a proper pelvic floor contraction and immediately got her started on the **Baby Bod**® Program.

I also suggested that she use a *Pelvic Floor Support Belt*^G for extra support during the day and talked to her about protecting her body from injury during the entire time she was breastfeeding and for three months after she stopped, for the reasons I explained above. I also taught her how she could safely use the elliptical machine, or bicycle or swim to get her cardio exercise and burn off calories. Under this regimen, her prolapse continued to get better.

Megan came back to see me three months after she stopped breastfeeding. We were able to upgrade her program to include higher-impact activities such as running, jumping, and playing tennis. Eventually, she was able to safely return to all her regular sports.

Keeping Yourself Safe

If you want to avoid a similar fate, look up from this page now and take a minute to think about your situation. How long has it been since you've had your baby? Is it less than three months? Are you still breastfeeding? And if you have stopped breastfeeding, has it been less than three months?

If you have answered *yes* to the last three questions, then you really have to baby your body for the time being. Take care to avoid **any activities that your body is not ready to handle**. Don't do *anything* that produces excess stress or strain on your body, such as moving heavy furniture, carrying heavy boxes or grocery bags, or returning to an exercise program that is too challenging for your current condition. If you have to lift, use good body mechanics and exhale upon exertion. There is more information on body mechanics and breathing techniques later on in the book. If you're a runner, tennis or volleyball player, or an enthusiast of any other sport, you'll also want to wait until your stability system is back to working order before you return to doing anything that could be jarring for your body.

---

^G The Pelvic Floor Support Belt supports the bottom of the pelvis. You can find one that I recommend at www.BabyBodBook.com. For more information on this, see either Chapter 8 or 9. The first one provides self-care advice for women who have had a vaginal birth; the second one provides self-care advice for women who have had a C-section. Please turn to the relevant chapter for you.

If you want to see how long you need to play it safe, try taking the two stability tests, the Straight Leg Raise Test and the Jumping Test. Your results will indicate if you are ready for more challenging, high-impact activities such as heavy lifting, jumping around a tennis court, or running. If you "pass" both tests, you may be able to return to high-impact activities even earlier than I suggested in the guidelines above. Even if you don't, you may be able to return to sports or perform more challenging activities earlier with the aid of a **Pelvic/SI Belt** or a **Pelvic Floor Support Belt**. In the second part of the Straight Leg Raise Test, I'll explain below how to tell if one of these belts can help improve your stability system. And in Chapters Eight and Nine, I will describe each belt in detail.

ASSESSING YOUR STABILITY SYSTEM

How do you know when your stability system is working optimally?

Use the two stability tests below, the **Straight Leg Raise Test** (both parts) and the **Jumping Test**, to evaluate your current condition and make an educated decision on when to return to more challenging activities like heavy lifting and strenuous or jarring sports. If you're pregnant, you can safely do both unless your healthcare provider has cautioned you against exercising. If you've had your baby, depending upon the kind of birth you had, you may be able to do these tests as early as two days after childbirth, and then repeat them on a weekly basis to assess your recovery. Mind you, these tests are not foolproof, but the results will give you the information you need to make the choice that is safest for your body in its present condition[H].

"Not so new" and older moms, I want you to do these too so you can see if your stability system has fully recovered from childbirth. If you have pain or incontinence now, the condition may have started when you were pregnant or in labor, even if it took a while to surface.

How do you know when your stability system is working optimally?

Take the tests on the right to evaluate your current condition.

[H] Ideally, all women would go for a postpartum check-up with a physical therapist or physiotherapist who has experience working with postpartum women. But until that becomes common practice in postnatal or antenatal care, here are two tests you can use to assess your recovery. If you do go for a physical therapy postnatal check-up, bring this book with you so you can use this program in conjunction with physical therapy treatment to recover as quickly as possible from childbirth.

I often see this in older moms who come in for treatment. That is how I came up with one of my favorite mantras: *"Once Postpartum, Always Postpartum®."*

Straight Leg Raise Test [11, 12, 13]

If you've had a baby, you may do this test as early as forty-eight hours after you had an *uncomplicated vaginal delivery.* Do your first check, and then continue rechecking on a weekly basis to monitor your progress.

If you've had a *C-section, a large vaginal or pelvic floor tear (3rd or 4th degree tear) or episiotomy,* however, you have to wait until after your six-week postpartum check-up and you have medical clearance to exercise. Then, after you do your first test, continue retesting on a weekly basis to monitor your progress.

The purpose of this self-test is to find out how well your core muscles are stabilizing your torso and to see if you are ready for more challenging exercises or activities. This test will also help you to see if you might benefit from using a Pelvic/SI Belt. There are two parts to this test: part one is done without using compression around your pelvis, and part two is done with compression, either by compressing your pelvis with your hands or by wearing a Pelvic/SI Belt.

The purpose of this self-test is to find out how well your core muscles are stabilizing your torso.

Straight Leg Raise Test – Part One (Without Compression):

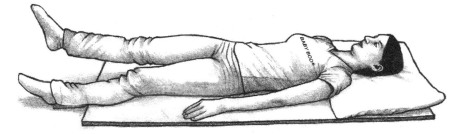

+ Lie on your back on a firm, flat surface.
+ Exhale gently as you slowly raise one leg about 6 to 8 inches. Notice how it feels. Then lower it.
+ Raise the other leg.
+ Record your results. *(see next page)*

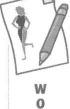

W
O
R
K
S
H
E
E
T

RESULTS		
Straight Leg Raise (Without Compression)	No?	Yes?
Does one leg feel heavier than the other?		
Do you feel like your pelvis is rocking while doing a straight leg raise?		
Do you notice any pain, and if so, record where (in the pelvis, abdomen or back).		
Do you notice a bulging in the middle of your belly?		

What did you notice? Please record and date your answers on the worksheet in Appendix A in the back of the book. This way, you'll be able to track your progress when you repeat this self-assessment test in the weeks ahead.

If you said **YES** to any of the questions above, it indicates that you need to work on recovering your core muscles before you return to challenging activities, like heavy lifting or participating in anything that requires jumping, jarring movements, or running. You will learn how to do this with the **Baby Bod® Program**, which will strengthen your body from the inside out.[1] Now take part two of this test to find out if you will benefit from using a Pelvic/SI Belt during the early part of this program.

Straight Leg Raise Test – Part Two (With Compression):

Now try this test by using your hands to produce a compressive force across your pelvis or by creating that compressive force by wearing a Pelvic/SI Belt. (Refer to Chapters Eight and Nine to learn more about Pelvic/SI Belts.) The compression from your hands or the belt will offer additional support if your stability system is compromised.

---

[1] To give credit where it's due, let me credit Australian physiotherapist Michelle Kenway, author of *Inside Out*, as the first person, to my knowledge, to talk about strengthening the body from the inside out.

Straight Leg Raise Test – Part Two (With Compression from Hands)

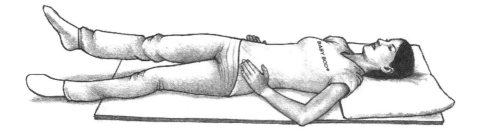

- Lie on your back on a firm, flat surface.
- Place both hands on the sides of your pelvis and squeeze them towards each other. Continue squeezing while raising your leg. (Refer to the illustration above.)
- Exhale gently as you slowly raise one leg about 6 to 8 inches. Notice how it feels. Then lower it.
- Raise the other leg.
- Record your results. *(see next page)*

Straight Leg Raise Test – Part Two (With Compression from Pelvic/SI Belt)

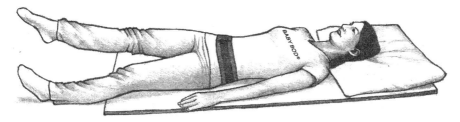

- Wrap the Pelvic/SI Belt around your pelvis. Make sure to wrap the belt tightly around the bony part of your pelvis and not around your waist.
- Lie on your back on a firm, flat surface. (Refer to the illustration above.)
- Exhale gently as you slowly raise one leg about 6 to 8 inches. Notice how it feels. Then lower it.
- Raise the other leg.
- Record your results. *(see next page)*

Compare your results to how it felt without the extra compression.

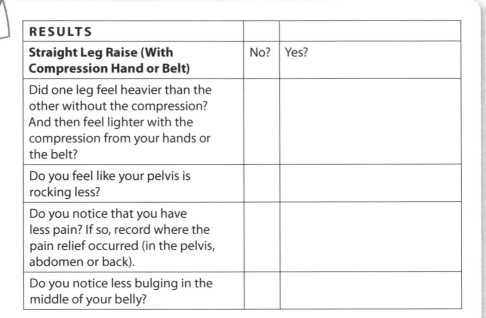

W O R K S H E E T

RESULTS		
Straight Leg Raise (With Compression Hand or Belt)	No?	Yes?
Did one leg feel heavier than the other without the compression? And then feel lighter with the compression from your hands or the belt?		
Do you feel like your pelvis is rocking less?		
Do you notice that you have less pain? If so, record where the pain relief occurred (in the pelvis, abdomen or back).		
Do you notice less bulging in the middle of your belly?		

Please record and date your answers on the worksheet in Appendix A. Continue repeating this test on a weekly basis to track your progress in the weeks ahead.

If you said **YES** to any of the questions above, it means that a Pelvic/SI Belt may be helpful in your recovery. You may use it for additional support over the next few months while you work on improving your stability system by following the **Baby Bod® Program**. Try to use the belt when performing more challenging activities such as standing for long periods of time, walking up inclines, stepping onto a ladder, or lifting heavy things.

How will I know if I passed the Straight Leg Raise Test?

Once you are able to do the straight leg test without using compression and do not feel one leg is heavier than the other, no longer feel pain, your pelvis does not rock, and your tummy does not bulge in the middle, you passed the test! It means that your stability system is in working order and you should be able to safely return to more challenging activities without any problems.

Note: *After you pass the Straight Leg Test, don't throw your Pelvic/ SI Belt away!* There may be times when you are overtired or fatigued or when you want to do something strenuous like increasing the amount of exercise you are doing, or you need to do some heavy lifting to get a household project done, or perhaps you need to climb on a ladder to paint. At times like these, you may find the extra compression offered by the Pelvic/SI Belt is helpful. I continue to use my Pelvic/SI Belt to prevent back pain when I travel and use it during my entire journey, even when I am sitting in the airplane. Some of my clients have found it useful to wear when they play sports, especially ones that require a lot of running or jumping.

Continue repeating this test on a weekly basis to track your progress in the weeks ahead.

JUMPING TEST: [J]

The purpose of this test is to see if you are ready for the more vigorous activities that require strong pelvic floor muscles. That includes activities like running and jumping or lifting heavy weights. Stop performing the test if you experience any pain, urine leakage, or the feeling that your organs are "bouncing" downwards against your pelvic floor. If you are pregnant, follow the same advice above. If you've had a baby, I usually recommend that women **wait at least three months after childbirth before performing this test.** If you are nursing, you may need to wait longer, until you are no longer under the influence of the "pregnancy hormones."

Record your results.

[J] Diane Edmonds, an Australian Physiotherapist developed this test. It is being reproduced here with her kind permission.

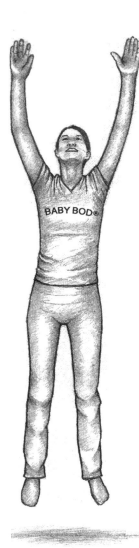

Jumping Test

+ Stand with your feet apart and with a full bladder.
+ Jump up and down (about 3 to 4 inches) 20 times, like jumping rope.
+ Then cough deeply at least three times.
+ Record your results.

What did you notice? Please record and date your answers on the worksheet in Appendix A to track your progress in the weeks ahead.

If you said **YES** to any of the questions in the chart provided below, you did not pass the Jumping Test. If you do feel increased pressure, or pain, or have leakage, consider waiting until you can pass this test before performing high-impact or jarring activities. That means you might not be ready to return to running, playing tennis, volleyball, heavy weight lifting, or swinging a kettlebell until you can pass the Jumping Test.

How Can I Return to Sports or Other Challenging Activities Before I Pass Both of these Tests?

I know—saying "please wait" won't do the trick for those of you who are chomping at the bit to get back to your pre-pregnancy workout routines earlier than the tests above indicate you should. So if you just can't wait, I urge you to consider using an *external pelvic support garment* to protect your pelvic floor along with a Pelvic/SI Belt (if you found it helpful above) while exercising. **There are many supportive undergarments readily available on the market, but I don't recommend many of them.** I will go into more detail about supportive garments and belts in Chapter Eight and Nine, and you can always check the **Baby Bod**® website store, at *www.BabyBodBook.com* to see what garments I recommend.

I have one final comment on "pregnancy hormones": Someday, we'll have more studies on the effects of hormones on postpartum

WORKSHEET

RESULTS		
Jumping Test (Wait until 3 Months Postpartum)	No?	Yes?
Do you feel any pain? If so, record where (pelvis, pelvic floor, abdomen, or back).		
Does it feel like your internal organs are "bouncing" up and down against your pelvic floor?		
Did you have any leakage of urine, feces or gas?		
Do you notice a bulging in the middle of your belly?		

Take the right steps to protect your body during the early postpartum phase after childbirth.

women. To date, we are not absolutely sure which hormones cause the connective tissue and ligaments to loosen up and how long the effects linger in the body after childbirth. [14, 5, 6] More research is definitely needed. If we had definitive answers to these questions, maybe more countries would start taking postpartum recovery much more seriously, and would come up with reasonable guidelines on how moms can protect their bodies during the vulnerable "connective-tissue laxity" period. Until then, I'd advise you to pay close attention to my suggestions.

* * *

These are the missing pieces I promised I would share. Aren't you glad you know them? Once you factor these in, it becomes clear how important it is to take the right steps to protect your body during the early postpartum phase after childbirth. You'll learn even more about why this is important in Chapter Seven, where I discuss in detail a number of disorders that are common—but not normal—in pregnant and postpartum women. Some of these conditions can be instigated or aggravated by doing too much, too soon.

[1] Panjabi MM. The Stabilizing System of the Spine. Part I. Function,Dysfunction, Adaptation, and Enhancement. *Journal of Spinal Disorders & Techniques*. 1992; 5(4):383-389. http://appliedspine.redhawk-tech.com/Medical-Professionals-and-Physicians/White-Papers/The_stabilizing_system_of_the_spine_part_1.pdf

[2] Lee D. Pelvic Stability & Your Core. Presented in whole or part at the: American Back Society Meeting – San Francisco 2005, BC Trial Lawyers Meeting – Vancouver 2005, Japanese Society of Posture & Movement Meeting – Tokyo 2006. http://dianelee.ca/articles/2PelvicStability&Yourcore.pdf

[3] Panjabi MM. The stabilizing system of the spine. Part II. Neural zone and instability hypothesis. *J Spinal Discord*. 1992; 5(4): 390-397. http://appliedspine.redhawk-tech.com/Medical-Professionals-and-Physicians/White-Papers/The_stabilizing_system_of_the_spine_part_2.pdf

[4] Lee D, Lee LJ. *The Pelvic Girdle, an Integration of Clinical Expertise and Research, 4th Edition*. Churchill Livingstone: Elsevier; 2011

[5] Marnach ML, Ramin KD, Ramsey PS, Song SW, Stensland JJ, An KN. Characterization of the relationship between joint laxity and maternal hormones in pregnancy. *Obstet Gynecol*. 2003 Feb; 101(2):331-5. doi: 10.1016/S0029-7844(02)02447 X.

[6] Vøllestad NK, Torjesen PA, Robinson HS. Association between the serum levels of relaxin and responses to the active straight leg raise test in pregnancy. *Man Ther*. 2012 Jun; 17(3):225-30. doi: 10.1016/j.math.2012.01.003. Epub 2012 Jan 30. http://www.ncbi.nlm.nih.gov/pubmed/22284767

[7] Sapsford R. Rehabilitation of pelvic floor muscles utilizing truck stabilization. *Manual Therapy*. 2004; 9:3-12.

[8] Lee D, Lee LJ. Stress Urinary Incontinence- A Consequence of Failed Load Transfer Through the Pelvis? Presented at: 5th World Interdisciplinary Congress on Low Back and Pelvic Pain;November 2004; Melbourne,Austrailia. http://s3.amazonaws.com/xlsuite_production/assets/1436205/StressUrinaryIncontinence.pdf

[9] Braekken IH, Majida M, Ellström EM, Holme IM, Bo K. Pelvic floor function is independently associated with pelvic organ prolapse. *BJOG*. 2009 Dec; 116(13):1706-14. doi: 10.1111/j.1471-0528.2009.02379.x.

[10] Hagen S, Stark D. Conservative prevention and management of pelvic organ prolapse in women. *Cochrane Database Syst Rev*. 2011 Dec 7; (12):CD003882. doi: 10.1002/14651858. CD003882.pub4.

[11] Mens JMA, Vleeming A, Snijders CJ, Stam HJ, Ginai AZ. The active straight leg raising test and mobility of the pelvic joints. *European Spine*. 1999; 8(6):468-73. doi: 10.1007/s005860050206

[12] Snijders CJ, Vleeming A, Stoeckart R. Transfer of lumbosacral load to iliac bones and legs. Part1: Biomechanics of selfbracing of the sacroiliac joints and its significance for treatment and exercise. *Clin Biomech*. 1993; 8(6):285-294. doi: 10.1016/0268-0033(93)90002-Y.

[13] Beales DJ, O'Sullivan PB, Briffa NK. Motor Control Patterns During an Active Straight Leg Raise in Chronic Pelvic Girdle Pain Subjects. *SPINE*.2009; 34(9):861–870. doi: 10.1097/BRS.0b013e318198d212

[14] Kristiansson P, Svardsudd K, von Schoultz B. Reproductive hormones and amino-terminal propeptide of type III procollagen in serum as early markers of pelvic pain during late pregnancy. *Am J Obst Gynecol*. 1999; 180(1 Pt 1):128-34. doi: 10.1016/S0002-9378(99)70162-6

Core Exercises: The Best Way to Flatten That "Mommy Tummy"

If you want to flatten your tummy after having a baby, you can't just exercise the muscles at the surface by doing sit-ups and other exercises targeting the abdominal muscles. After childbirth, you have to restore your core muscles first.

Many moms don't know this, which is why they can't quite flatten that tummy, no matter how hard they try. Some well-intentioned moms do the wrong exercises and make things worse. Or they sabotage themselves even when they're not exercising, completely unaware that the way they breathe or carry their body makes that "Mommy Tummy" bulge out even more.

In this chapter, I am going to explain how your *inner core muscles* work and how they interact with your *outer core muscles*—before and after you give birth. And then we're going to look at the most effective way to restore the core muscles to optimal function once again, which *has* to happen to flatten your tummy and keep it flat.

A Brief Review

As I said earlier in the anatomy chapter, the *core muscles* are the ones that are deepest in the body; they form the "*inner muscle system.*" In that chapter, I identified each of the four core muscles and explained that they function as a group. We're going to build on that knowledge now. And then we'll look at how they work in coordination with the outer abdominal muscles to flatten your tummy and to stabilize your torso during all your everyday activities.

The front and back of the core muscles wrap around your internal organs and spine. The front is made up of the *transverse abdominis muscle* and the back is formed by the *multifidus muscles*. At the top

Some well-intentioned moms do the wrong exercises and make things worse.

is the *diaphragm* and on the bottom are the *pelvic floor muscles*; together, they form the top and base of the core muscles. (Please refer back to Chapter Four for more detailed information on these muscles.) Notice in the illustration below how these muscles "wrap" around the internal organs and form the "core" of your body. The core muscles form a "closed system," surrounding everything inside your tummy.

CORE MUSCLES

Core muscles encase the internal organs and sit inside of the pelvis.

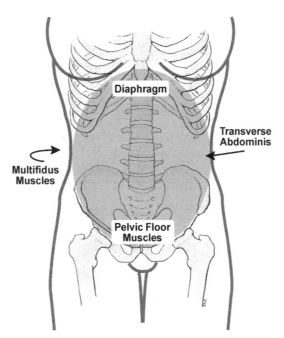

LifeART and MediClip image copyright 2013 Wolters Kluwer Health, Inc. Lippincott Williams & Wilkins. All rights reserved.

It's probably easiest to imagine this group of muscles as a "balloon" that encases your internal organs.[A] This balloon sits deep inside your pelvis and just under your rib cage. So if there is pressure placed on the balloon, you will see the balloon change shape. For example, if you press down on the top of the "core balloon," all the abdominal organs will be pressed downwards towards the pelvic floor. Looking at the illustration above will make this clearer.

[A] The "core" balloon" is the unique idea of Julie Wiebe, PT, www.JulieWiebePT.com.

KEY DIFFERENCES IN THE "OUTER" AND "INNER" MUSCLES

Now that you're familiar with the core muscles, let's pull back a bit and compare both layers of muscle—the *inner* and the *outer muscle systems* in your body. The truth is, you need to use both of these muscle groups—the *outer* and the *inner*—to get back in shape.

They each perform somewhat differently. The outer muscles function as the *"movers,"* while the inner core muscles serve as the *"holders."* You need to understand these differences so that you fully understand the role of each of the steps in the **Baby Bod® Program**.

With the **outer muscles**, the *"movers,"* you can see muscle definition easily after you lift weights. I like to tell my clients to think of the outer muscles as the same type of muscles Popeye flexes after he eats his can of spinach. You can also think of these outer muscles as the "pumping iron" muscles, because these are the muscles that you strengthen when you lift weights.

These muscles lie on the outermost parts of your body and are responsible for allowing you to move your arm when you reach forward to pick up a package, or move your legs to walk down the street. The muscles that form that six-pack, the *rectus abdominis*, are considered outer muscles because they are responsible for bending your torso.

Contrast that with the **inner core muscle**, *or the "holders."* These muscles hold your spine and torso together while you move, help to hold your internal organs in place, and play an important role in flattening your tummy. They form a "corset of support" and are an essential part of the stability system we discussed in the last chapter.

Here's the other key difference: You *can't* strengthen *inner core muscles* with traditional mainstream or "pumping-iron" type exercises; you need to do specific exercises to activate them or wake them up when they are not working up to par. [1, 2, 3] Another important point that many exercise enthusiasts do not understand is that you can, however, influence how well your core muscles function by the way you align your body during movement [4] and by the way you breathe. [1] That means you *need to use the correct form and breathing techniques when doing core exercises,* something I will teach you in the chapters ahead.

MUSCLE "BALANCE" IS IMPORTANT – A TEAM APPROACH[1, 5, 6, 7]

The core muscles "team up" with the outer muscles to support your body as you move around. There is an ideal relationship between the outer muscles and inner core muscles. In short, they're meant to work together in a *balanced, coordinated* way to help you accomplish whatever you're doing that requires movement.

When you go to lift your baby out of his or her crib, for instance, your inner core muscles work to hold your spine and pelvis together while your outer muscles work to lift the baby. If your core muscles are working properly when you lift your infant out of the crib, your arms can move more efficiently because they have a stable base to move upon.

If the inner and outer muscles do not work in balance and in coordination with each other, you will not have this base of support and you will lose the *stabilizing hold* from the core muscles. Sometimes the outer muscles can become overdeveloped and take over the work of the inner core muscle system, causing a loss in stability. That's a problem. Imagine trying to reach for something on a high shelf if the middle part of your body were made of Jell-O. Not very stable, is it?

How might the outer muscles become overdeveloped? By doing the **wrong** types of exercises, and yes, even by the way you carry yourself throughout the day. Both of these can interfere with this balance and prevent the inner and outer muscles from working in balance and coordination with each other.

I bet you are now scratching your head and wondering, "What exercises can I use to flatten my tummy?" Don't worry; I made it easy for you! The exercises I have developed in the **Baby Bod® Program** are carefully designed to prevent you from developing muscle imbalances and to teach you how to move in the most efficient way during all your daily activities. This program shows you the RIGHT way to strengthen your core after you've given birth.

How the Core Muscles SHOULD Work [1, 2, 3, 8, 9, 10, 11]

When the core muscles are functioning optimally, they contract automatically to prepare you for movement. The core muscles

The core muscles literally "hold you together" so you can move from a place of stability.

literally "hold you together" so you can move from a place of stability. Right after the core muscles contract, the outer muscles—the "movers"—normally spring into action.

Let's say you go to lift a heavy package, for instance. If everything is working as it should, you automatically exhale and your core muscles get the message to contract to support your body. Your pelvic floor muscles lift upwards, your inner abdominal muscles draw in your tummy, and your deep back muscles draw in to support the spine, forming a solid, "balloon-shaped corset" of support inside your torso. (This all happens in a nanosecond!) Then the outer muscles in your legs bend to bring you closer to the package on the floor. As you continue, the muscles in your upper body reach your arms toward the package and continue to contract as you lift the package up. End result: You accomplish the lift with power and grace, without injury to yourself.

How Breathing Influences Your Core Muscles and Intra-Abdominal Pressure [1, 10]

How well both groups of muscles in your abdomen work together as a team to stabilize your torso and flatten your tummy is determined by the amount of pressure you have inside your belly, which is known as *intra-abdominal pressure*. This pressure system is influenced by the way you *breathe* and *the coordination of both layers of abdominal muscles*. If you want a stable core and a flat tummy, this *internal pressure system* needs to work in balance with the core muscles and the outer abdominal muscles. To do this, you need to learn how to breathe correctly to keep the pressure just right, as I will explain on the next page.

What happens to your core muscles when you breathe?

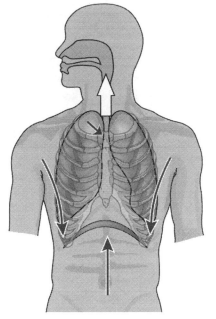

Inhalation

When you inhale, the diaphragm
contracts and moves downwards.
This increases the pressure inside the
belly (intra-abdominal pressure).

Exhalation

When you exhale, the diaphragm
relaxes which decreases
intra-abdominal pressure.

In the anatomy chapter, I described the diaphragm as a large
dome-shaped muscle that separates your stomach and other internal
organs from the lungs. (Please refer to the illustration in Chapter
Four.) During normal *inhalation*, your rib cage expands and the
dome of the diaphragm flattens to make more room in the chest so
the lungs can fill up with air. As the diaphragm flattens, it pushes
down on the abdominal organs and exerts downward pressure into
your abdominal cavity, which *increases intra-abdominal pressure*.
This creates a multidirectional force, which pushes the pelvic floor
downwards and the lower abdominal muscles outwards.

In order to stabilize your body and keep your tummy flat during
inhalation, the lower tummy and pelvic floor muscles need to work
harder to match this increase in pressure or else you will have a
failure in the system. If the muscles are working as a team, this

usually is not a problem. If this pressure is too strong or stays elevated for longer periods of time, however, it could strain and eventually fatigue these muscles, which means you could end up with an undesirable bulge in your lower tummy (AKA "Mommy Tummy") and a droopy pelvic floor. It could also lead to back and pelvic pain and urine leakage.

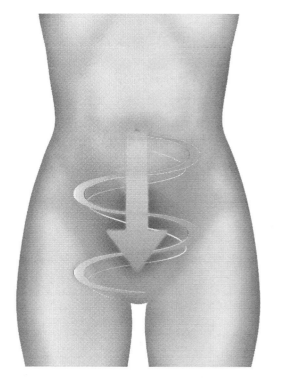

Andrea Danti/Shutterstock.com

Intra-Abdominal Pressure

When intra-abdominal pressure increases, it can lead to straining the connective tissue and muscles in the lower abdomen and pelvic floor area.

When you exhale, your diaphragm moves back up and away from your abdominal organs and the lungs deflate. As you continue to exhale, the intra-abdominal pressure *decreases*, the pelvic floor muscles move upwards, and your abdominal muscles move inwards to support your organs. *The brain actually sends a message to the core muscles to contract during exhalation.* Since there is a decrease in intra-abdominal pressure, the core and abdominal muscles do not need to work as hard to maintain a flat tummy. In essence, **when you exhale, your body naturally becomes more stable because it is *easier* for the core muscles to work and the brain "encourages" them to contract and support your body.**

When your body is functioning optimally, this is a *normal breathing cycle* and you are able to maintain stability and a flat tummy whether you are inhaling or exhaling. Your body uses breathing to help regulate the pressure in your abdomen, which has a direct effect on your ability to stabilize your torso. Problems can arise if you lose coordination of this entire system and you inhale at the wrong time or hold your breath for prolonged periods of time, as I will explain shortly.

How Breathing Influences the Core Muscles	
Inhalation	**Exhalation**
Increases intra-abdominal pressure.	Decreases intra-abdominal pressure.
Makes it harder for the core muscles to work.	Encourages the core muscles to work.
Places extra pressure on your lower tummy and pelvic floor muscles.	Encourages the abdominal muscles to flatten your tummy.
Requires the muscles to work as a coordinated team to maintain stability and a flat tummy.	Increases stability and a flat tummy.

How to Feel Intra-Abdominal Pressure

To help you feel this pressure in your body so you can remember it, I want you to try the following and record your results in your worksheet: Place a hand on your tummy, take a big breath in, and hold it. Do you feel your abdominal muscles stretching and your belly popping outwards? That means that the pressure inside your belly has increased. Good. Now, exhale.

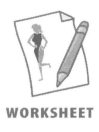

WORKSHEET

Now try this: Place a hand on your belly and gently exhale, as if you are cleaning a pair of sunglasses. Make sure to empty all the air in your lungs. When you finish exhaling, do you feel as if your abdominal muscles are working more and pulling in your tummy a bit? When you exhale, the deepest layer of abdominal muscle and all the other core muscles should naturally contract to form a corset of internal support and flatten your tummy.

The take away here is that when you *inhale*, the result is increased intra-abdominal pressure. That means that your pelvic floor and lower abdominal muscles need to work harder and meet that pressure to maintain stability and to keep your tummy flat. If the muscles are not able to meet that pressure, you end up with a bulge in your tummy and lose the central support system normally offered by the core and outer abdominal muscles. When you *exhale*, the opposite occurs; the intra-abdominal pressure *decreases* and the core muscles are encouraged to work to stabilize your torso and flatten your tummy. (This is the reason why I will ask you to exhale or count out loud when you are doing the **Baby Bod® exercises**.)

Guess what happens when you hold your breath?

If you inhale and hold your breath, the pelvic floor and abdominal muscle will need to work **overtime** to meet this pressure. If you develop a habit of holding your breath for prolonged periods of time when you exert yourself, it can eventually lead to muscle strain and fatigue, and that, in turn, can cause you to develop core muscle weakness, pain and/or incontinence.

Stop Breath-Holding Behavior!

After childbirth, your core muscles and outer abdominal muscles are stretched out and weak. This leads to a failure in the stability system, and you lose the normal corset of support you had prior to becoming pregnant. To make up for this, you may naturally try to stabilize or "brace" your abdomen by holding your breath to make yourself stronger. Doing this day in and day out can lead to trouble and you can develop pain or start leaking urine every time you pick up your baby.

The advice I give my clients is to try to stop *"breath-holding behavior."* In other words, remember to exhale whenever you exert yourself, even if you're doing something as simple as getting up from a chair. This will decrease the pressure in your abdomen, rather than exacerbate that "Mommy Tummy." You don't need to exhale a lot— just enough to match your activity. When you pick up your newborn baby out of a crib, for instance, try exhaling as if you're cleaning off sunglasses. When you lift a heavy pot off of the stove, try exhaling a little more deeply. If you need to pick up a heavy suitcase, try exhaling even harder to prevent straining your abdominal and pelvic floor muscles. Try to become more aware of how you breathe during your everyday activities and when you are exercising. You may discover that you have developed a tendency to hold your breath as a way to get through your day. Each time you catch yourself holding your breath, STOP and try to exhale when you exert yourself. I will teach you how to change this behavior as you progress with the **Baby Bod® Program**.

* * *

Do you hold your breath when you do the following?

Try doing each of the activities listed in the chart below and record your results in your worksheet.

If you answered YES, try to exhale instead of holding your breath. And remember that the amount you need to exhale should match the level of the activity you are engaging in.

Baby Bod® Tip:
Don't hold your breath to manage a load; instead exhale upon exertion.

W O R K S H E E T

Do you hold your breath when doing the following?	No?	Yes?
Pick up or carry your baby?		
Pick up heavy packages or the stroller?		
Reach for something on the top shelf in the grocery store?		
Push a vacuum or heavy door?		
Pull something heavy?		
Lift a pot of pasta off the stove?		
Play sports like hitting a tennis ball?		

Breathing Techniques When You Exercise

Breathing correctly is essential when you are doing the exercises. It is VERY IMPORTANT to follow *EXACTLY* the instructions I give about breathing while you are doing these exercises. Pay attention when I instruct you to **EXHALE** or **COUNT OUT LOUD** in the exercise instructions. Counting out loud will keep your air passages open and prevent building up extra pressure in your belly. Counting out loud makes it impossible to hold your breath. Over time, if you hold your breath while doing these exercises, it can cause more harm than good.

How Body Alignment Influences Core Muscles [1, 2, 8, 9]

As you've seen, the way you breathe makes a big difference in how your core muscles function. The same is true for the way you carry yourself during your everyday activities and when you exercise. Let's call this "body alignment" rather than posture. *Core muscles work best when you use good alignment.* This is important to keep in mind if you want to flatten that "Mommy Tummy."

Correct alignment can improve the ability of the core muscles to flatten your tummy. If you carry yourself incorrectly, it can interfere with how well the core muscles work. Few women realize this, but it's true nonetheless: if your body alignment is off, it can cause your belly to bulge. It can also cause or worsen conditions such as back and pelvic pain and or incontinence.

Look at the illustration below to see how much better you can look when you correct your alignment by stacking your rib cage over the pelvis, something I will teach you to do later on in the chapter on alignment. The woman in the illustration on the right has corrected her alignment. Her profile looks slimmer because her core muscles are working more efficiently to flatten her tummy.

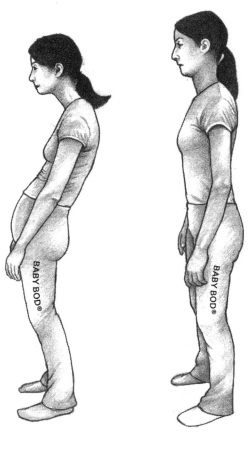

Correct alignment will help the core muscles to work optimally and to make your tummy look flatter too.

* * *

Well, that's it for the quick anatomy lesson on core muscles. When they are working optimally, they flatten your tummy and create the stability you need for smooth and safe movement. As I explained, the two factors that most influence how well the core muscles work are your: 1) alignment, and 2) breathing technique.

Now we're going to look at how pregnancy and childbirth affect the core muscles. Once you understand this, you'll realize why you can't flatten that tummy just by doing exercises that target the abdominal muscles.

Why You Need to Retrain Your Core Muscles After Childbirth

It's no secret that pregnancy causes certain muscles to stretch—a LOT. Once the muscles stretch past a certain point to accommodate the growing child, it disrupts the connection between the brain and those muscles, "deactivating" the affected muscles. Think about what happens when you turn off a light switch. That's analogous to what happens when muscles get de-activated. Once that happens, they "forget" how to effectively coordinate their actions with those of your outer muscles, as they would normally do to stabilize your body.

Here's the real kicker: After you give birth, those muscles don't always "turn back on" on their own. It's up to **you** to help them by doing special exercises designed to re-activate or retrain the core muscles, such as the ones I will teach you in the **Preliminary Phase** of this program. Mainstream exercises—even those that are supposed to work your tummy—won't do it. Studies have shown that you need to do *specific* exercises—with the right form and timing—to fully *reactivate* the core muscles to work in a coordinated manor with your outer abdominal muscles. These "training" exercises repair the communication between the brain and the core muscles so that the sequence of muscle activation happens as it should.

You **can't** skip this step and expect great results. *In fact, if you try to strengthen the core muscles without retraining them first, you'll reinforce the existing problem of impaired function, which* *will prevent you from flattening your tummy. This can eventually lead to back and pelvic pain, and/or incontinence.*

Two Stages of Exercises

That's why the **Baby Bod® Program** takes a two-part approach. You'll **train** the core muscles first in the **Preliminary Phase Exercises**, where you will learn how to "flick the switch" back on to your core muscles to remind them how to work in coordination with your outer abdominal muscles. Once you have learned how to "activate" your core muscles, you can proceed to the second stage, which focuses on **strengthening**. *Most moms need to do the types of core exercises in the sequence I will teach you in the Baby Bod® Program.*

Older or more experienced moms, this is why you need to do one week of the **Preliminary Phase Exercises** before you go onto the advanced exercises and to continue doing them a few times a week while you are doing the more advanced, strengthening exercises. Yes, they *are* necessary. They'll help you restore optimal functioning to the core muscles that never fully recovered from pregnancy.

I'm a prime example. I suffered from postpartum incontinence for longer than I should have because I didn't know there was a solution. I tried traditional pelvic floor treatment that included using a biofeedback machine to retrain my pelvic floor muscle for several months, and it didn't work. I was religious about doing Kegel exercises three times a day, and it did not stop the leakage I experienced when I coughed, sneezed, laughed and jumped. After I developed this program and practiced it, I no longer had that problem.

You must re-train (or activate) your core muscles prior to doing strengthening exercises

* * *

Four Keys to Recovering Your Core:

If you want to lose your "Mommy Tummy," here is a list of guidelines you must follow to re-train and then strengthen your core muscles.

1. **You *can't* strengthen core muscles *with traditional "mainstream exercises."*** *Core muscles require two levels of exercises to get them back into shape after childbirth.* You must *re-train* (or activate) your core muscles prior to doing strengthening exercises. Please follow the sequence provided for you in the **Baby Bod® Program.**

2. **You have to breathe correctly.** As I mentioned earlier in this chapter, breathing helps to control intra-abdominal pressure. When you are doing **Baby Bod® exercises**, please be sure to follow EXACTLY the instructions I give about breathing while you are doing the exercises. Pay attention when I instruct you to **EXHALE** or **COUNT OUT LOUD.**

3. **You have to use the right form—and by that I mean to get your body in the best alignment possible when exercising and during all of your everyday activities.** When your bones and muscles are in the right alignment, your muscles—including the ones that hold in your tummy— work most efficiently. To help you get your alignment right, I'm going to teach you a simple six-step series, the **Baby Bod® Alignment Check**, in Chapter Eleven. And I will remind you about alignment when I teach you the exercises.

4. **Don't do exercises that are too challenging for your current condition**, no matter how tempted you may be. If you want a flat tummy, follow the sequential order as directed in this program.

In Summary

In the **Baby Bod® Program**, you will learn exercises that will *strengthen you from the inside out*. There are two stages in this program. First you will learn how to activate or train your core muscles the correct way, while using the right form, timing and breathing techniques. Then you will proceed to stage two in your recovery and do strengthening exercises.

Let's move on. In the next chapter, we'll look at some medical conditions commonly associated with pregnancy and birth and what you can do on your own, or with professional care to prevent, relieve, or alleviate them.

Let's move on.

[1] Hodges PW, Sapsford R, Pengel LH. Postural and Respiratory Functions of the Pelvic Floor Muscles. *Neurology and Urodyamics*. 2007; 26(3):362-371. doi: 10.1002/nau.20232

[2] Sapsford R. Rehabilitation of pelvic floor muscles utilizing trunk stabilization. *Manual Therapy*. 2004 Feb; 9(1):3-12.

[3] Hodges PW, Richardson CA. Potential risk of low back injury with limb movement at varying speeds with special reference to muscular stabilisation of the spine. *Scand J Med Sa Sports*. 1995; 5(4):262.

[4] Carriere B. Interdependence of posture and the pelvic floor. *The pelvic floor*. New York: Georg Thieme Verlag; 2006; 68–8.

[5] Hodges PW, Richardson CA. Inefficient muscular stabilization of the lumbar spine associated with low back pain. A motor control evaluation of transversus abdominis. *Spine*.1996; 21(22): 2640-50. http://www.udel.edu/PT/manal/spinecourse/Exercise/hodgesinefficientstab.pdf

[6] Hodges PW. Core stability exercise in chronic low back pain. *Orthop Clin North Am*. 2003;34(2): 245-54. http://nucre.com/Artigos%20-%20Coluna/Core_stability_exercise.pdf

[7] Hodges P W, Cholewicki J. Functional control of the spine. In: Vleeming A, Mooney V, Stockhart R, eds. *Movement, Stability & Lumbopelvic Pain: Integration of Research and Therapy*. 2nd ed. Edinburgh,UK: Churchill Livingstone; 2007: 489-512.

[8] Lee D, Lee LJ. Stress Urinary Incontinence- A Consequence of Failed Load Transfer Through the Pelvis? Presented at: 5th World Interdisciplinary Congress on Low Back and Pelvic Pain;November 2004; Melbourne,Austrailia. http://s3.amazonaws.com/xlsuite_production/assets/1436205/StressUrinaryIncontinence.pdf

[9] Sahrmann SA. *Diagnosis and Treatment of Movement Impairment Syndromes*. Arbor, Michigan:Mosby; 2001

[10] Lee LJ, McLaughlin L. Stability, continence and breathing: the role of fascia following pregnancy and delivery. *J Bodyw Mov Ther*. 2008 Oct; 12(4):333-48. doi: 10.1016/j.jbmt.2008.05.003.

[11] Lee D. Core Training vs. Strengthening- What is the Difference and Why Does it Matter? Diane Lee & Associates Physiotherapy. http://dianelee.ca/article-core-training-versus-strengthening.php

CHAPTER SEVEN

What Momma Never Told You About Childbirth

The process of giving birth to a new life is not without some risk. It can—and in certain cases does—result in not-so-fun changes that can ultimately lead to a diagnosable disorder. In this chapter, I'm going to help you assess whether the changes you've experienced are normal and will heal on their own, or whether they require more intensive self-care or professional care.

So let's jump right in. Yes, we'll be looking at things that might make you squeamish, such as muscle separation, leaking urine, pelvic pain, and organs protruding out of your lady parts (known in medical parlance as *diastasis recti, incontinence, pelvic pain and pelvic organ prolapse*, respectively). There's no way around it; we've got to go there so you have the info you need—in case you need it—to bring about full recovery after childbirth.

Ready or not, let's get started!

DIASTASIS RECTI

Dia...what?

Did you ever wonder why so many moms still look pregnant several months or even years after they deliver their baby? It's likely these moms have **diastasis recti**, the medical condition I described in Chapter Four. Normally, the *linea alba* is taut. It serves to anchor the two rectus abdominal muscle strips in place, allowing them to remain relatively parallel to each other, on either side of your belly button.

In diastasis recti, however, the rectus abdominal muscle strips—the so-called "six-pack" muscles at the abdomen's surface—spread apart. It's not that there's a true cut or a tear, but a spreading out

Ever wonder why so many moms still look pregnant several months or even years after they deliver their baby?

of the connective tissue that joins the right and left halves of this muscle. These two muscle strips don't directly attach to each other; they attach to a band of connective tissue called the *linea alba*, which joins them. (Please see below.)

DIASTASIS-RECTI

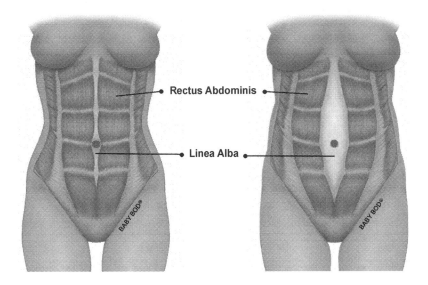

The hormones produced during pregnancy will make this connective tissue, the linea alba, looser and less firm, which will make it easier for the belly to expand to accommodate the uterus as it increases in size along with the baby. (Again, please see the illustration above.)

The spreading out of the connective tissue is a normal occurrence as the baby grows and usually resolves on its own. In most women, the connective tissue stiffens up and closes the gap between the two sides of the rectus abdominis muscle within the first six weeks after childbirth. Studies show, however, that this does *not* automatically "close" in about one-third of women with this condition,[1] leaving them with the dreaded "Mommy Tummy."

When the linea alba stretches so much that it can no longer hold the two sides of the muscle in place, the muscles are not able to contract in a straight line. Instead of pulling the tummy in, they form a "bow" shape around the belly button, which makes the belly bulge out in a dome shape in the middle of the tummy. Yup, that is a "Mommy Tummy." Not a pretty picture, I know.

Diastasis recti is fairly common in new mothers. If you have this condition, the earlier you know about it, the better. Studies have shown that women who have a diastasis recti are more likely to develop lower back pain, incontinence, and pelvic organ prolapse, conditions you definitely want to stop in their tracks. [2, 3, 4, 5, 6] There are definitely things you can do to promote healing and, at the very least, prevent it from getting worse. If you ignore it, however, you can unknowingly make the condition worse.

Even if you don't have diastasis recti now, you need to be aware of the condition and watchful. Studies show that it can develop years after you give birth. [3]

If you have diastasis recti, the earlier you know about it, the better.

Assessing Yourself – Measuring the Gap

If you think you might have diastasis recti, it's pretty simple to test yourself. Basically, you will be using your fingers to determine how wide the separation or the gap is. If you have *more than two fingers of separation*, it is considered problematic. [2] After you do the Diastasis Recti Test (below), please do the Straight Leg Raise Test that follows.

Diastasis Recti Test

You may do this test as early as forty-eight hours after you have a vaginal delivery. Make sure to record your results in your worksheets. Once you do your first check, go ahead with the program and then use this test to recheck yourself once a week.

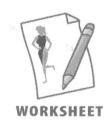

WORKSHEET

If you've had a **C-section, a large vaginal** or **pelvic floor tear** (Grade 3 or 4) [A] or an **episiotomy**, however, please wait until you have medical clearance to exercise after your six-week checkup before doing this test. Once you have reached the six-week benchmark and you have been told you can resume normal activities, start doing this test on a weekly basis.

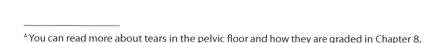

[A] You can read more about tears in the pelvic floor and how they are graded in Chapter 8, the self-care chapter on vaginal delivery.

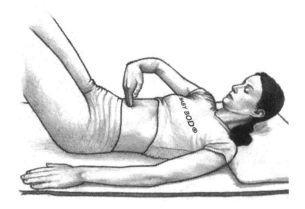

Here's how to do it:

+ Lie on a firm, flat surface. Use a pillow to support your head and bend your knees so that your feet are flat on the floor.
+ Relax your tummy muscles.
+ Place one hand on your belly as follows: First, point your fingers down towards your tummy and hold your hand horizontally so you can see the palm or inside of your hand. Keep your fingers together and place them about 2 inches (5cm) above your belly button. (Please refer to the illustration above if this is not clear to you.)
+ *Gently* push your fingers down into your abdomen and keep them there as you lift your head up. *(If this is painful, use less pressure.)*
+ Keep your shoulders on the floor or mat; do not perform a crunch by lifting your chest up.
+ Do you feel a soft space between your muscles? If so, how far apart is it? Measure this by how many fingers you can fit in the soft spot. Is it one finger width? Two fingers' width? Three fingers' width or more?
+ Feel for the separation or gap in two areas:
  1. Just above the belly button (about 2 inches or 5cm), and
  2. Just below the belly button (about 1 inch or 2.5cm)

What did you find after doing your test? Please record and date your findings on the worksheet. Write down how many finger widths of separation you found. If you have diastasis recti, this will help you track your progress when you re-test for diastasis recti in the weeks ahead.

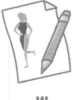

WORKSHEET

Diastasis Recti Questions	Your Answers
Do you feel a soft spot between your muscles?	
How many fingers can you fit into the soft spot? Is it one finger width? Two fingers' width? Three fingers' width?	
Feel for the separation about 2 inches above the belly button. Write down how far apart it is:	
Feel for the separation about 1 inch below the belly button. Write down how far apart it is:	

Straight Leg Raise Test:

Right after you test yourself for diastasis recti, it's good to do the Straight Leg Raise Test that was described in Chapter Five. (Make sure to do part one and part two of this test.) If you can pass the Straight Leg Raise Test without your belly bulging or your pelvis wobbling, and/or with both legs feeling equal in weight when you lift them, then you probably have good stability. That means even if you have a diastasis recti, the soft tissue in between the two rectus abdominal muscles are firm enough to hold the muscles in place and your core muscles are working optimally. Therefore, your stability system is in good working order. Some women are able to recover their core strength and stability by doing the right exercises, like the ones you will learn in **Baby Bod**®, even if they have a diastasis.

WORKSHEET

If you do not pass the test, consider using a Pelvic/SI Belt for extra support (see Chapter Eight or Nine) and continue progressing with the **Baby Bod® Program** and testing your stability on a weekly basis.

How to Care for Diastasis Recti

First, you want to **prevent diastasis recti from getting worse** by protecting your abdomen during the entire time that your connective tissue remains under the influence of the "pregnancy hormones," which make these tissues looser than normal. (As I said in Chapter Five, that period of vulnerability could last for up to three months after you give birth, or, if you are breastfeeding, the entire time you are nursing and up until three months after you stop breastfeeding.) During this time, there are some activities you may want to avoid to protect your abdomen.

Things to Avoid When You Have Diastasis Recti:

1. **Avoid strenuous activities or exercises that place strain on the belly.** Believe it or not, just holding your breath when you get up from a chair, carry your stroller, or lift your child can increase internal pressure in your belly, and this pressure will push the linea alba outwards, causing it to spread more. Engaging in activities that **increase the internal pressure in your belly** for prolonged periods of time or that are so challenging they cause you to hold your breath will place more strain on the linea alba and force the muscles to separate more. If you do have to engage in an activity that requires exertion, make sure to EXHALE as you perform the activity.

2. **Avoid "jackknife behavior,"** such as getting up from bed or up from the floor as if you are doing a sit-up. Instead, learn the log roll and push-up sideways technique I describe in the next two chapters on self-care and use those techniques. (Chapter Eight is for those of you who had a vaginal birth; the one after that, Chapter Nine, is for those of you who have had a C-section. Please go to the chapter that pertains to you.)

3. If you exercise, you also want to **avoid sit-ups and sports that require a lot of core strength** until your diastasis is closed or you have restored your core strength. Every time you do a sit-up, you will increase the amount of internal pressure in your belly and risk further separation.[B] A large amount of stability and core strength is required in certain sports, like tennis or golf, and if you get back to your game too early (before you recover your core strength), it can place excess strain on the connective tissue and make a diastasis worse. Both the Straight Leg Raise Test and the Jumping Test in Chapter Five should help you determine if you are ready to safely return to these activities.

4. **Avoid stiff or tight elastic abdominal binders**. These will eventually cause the abdominal muscles to become weaker if you use them for prolonged periods of time. Even though the binders have become trendy, they will NOT help you get rid of your "Mommy Tummy," and they actually make it worse in the long run.[C] In rare cases, an abdominal binder may be medically necessary, like during the week or two after a C-section. In those cases, listen to your doctor or physical therapist and use one. (But try not to use a binder for long periods of time.)

5. **Prevent constipation**. When someone is constipated, they tend to take in a deep breath and try to push that bowel movement out. That pushing causes an increase in intra-abdominal pressure, which can put further strain on the linea alba, causing the strips of rectus muscle to separate further. Pushing also places a lot of strain on the pelvic floor muscles and connective tissue in the pelvic region, which could further weaken this area. (Please read the tips below on how to prevent constipation.)

[B] Read more about the negative effects of sit-ups in Chapter 10.

[C] Read more about abdominal binders in Chapter 8 or 9.

Things to Do: Caring for Diastasis Recti

1. Wear a pair of the **long-waisted shorts with medical grade compression** during the day for at least a few months after childbirth. DO NOT wear tight shape-wear as a substitute. If you do not want to wear a compression garment, you may want to try using the **Baby Bod® Abdominal Wrap**. (You can read more about compression garments and the wrap in Chapter Eight and Nine.)

2. Try wearing a Pelvic/SI Belt to add a little more support. (If you didn't take the Straight Leg Raise Test in Chapter Five, please turn back and take the test now. It will help you determine whether the Pelvic/SI Belt will work best for you.)

3. Use **good body mechanics** to prevent increasing the internal pressure in your belly, which will cause further separation of the muscles. (For excellent tips, see Chapter Seventeen, "Get Your **Baby Bod®** On All Day Long.")

4. Try the simple **Diastasis Recti Massage technique** you will find in the next two chapters. (You'll find these in Chapter Eight for women who had a vaginal delivery and in Chapter Nine for women who had a Cesarean section delivery. Please go to the chapter that pertains to you.)

5. **Exhale** when you exert yourself to prevent pressure from building up inside your abdomen. Make sure the amount you exhale matches the level of activity. When you go to pick up a small object, like a toy from the floor, exhale softly. When you try to lift a heavy grocery bag, exhale more deeply. Try to not to hold your breath when lifting, pushing and pulling.

6. Prevent **constipation** by eating a good diet with plenty of fiber. Drink a lot of water and try doing the **Constipation Self-Massage** that you will find in the next two chapters on self-care.

(Please choose the chapter that pertains to you.) Also, use the good toileting habits that are discussed later in this chapter.

7. **Continue to do the Diastasis Recti and the Straight Leg Raise self-tests** once a week to check on your progress—or lack of progress.

8. **Do the Baby Bod® exercises** in this book.

How long you need to protect your abdomen after childbirth depends on whether you are breastfeeding your baby. One of the main factors that could be preventing a diastasis recti from closing up is the *lingering effect of the "pregnancy hormones"*—something I discussed in depth in Chapter Five. Here is what I recommend:

+ If you are **bottle-feeding your child**, I recommend that you continue to take precautions to protect your belly during the first three months after delivering your baby.
+ If you are **nursing your baby**, however, please continue to take precautions to protect your belly during the entire time you are breastfeeding and for a few months after you wean your baby.

How long will I need to continue testing for a diastasis? Fortunately, many women with diastasis recti recover fully with time. Checking yourself regularly for diastasis—or for the progress you are making or *not* making—is good preventative care. It is a good idea to **continue to perform the Diastasis Recti Test and the Straight Leg Raise Test during the entire time that your body may be under the influence of the "pregnancy hormones."** (That means for three months for moms who bottle-feed, and for breastfeeding moms during the entire time you are nursing and for three months after you wean your baby.) If you have diastasis recti, frequent testing on a weekly basis will also keep it at the forefront of your mind and make it more likely that you'll remember to avoid activities that can increase pressure on the diastasis and make it worse.

When should I seek professional help? If you do have diastasis recti, report it to your physician or nurse midwife. You can try progressing with the **Baby Bod® Program** to see if doing the right exercises—and giving your body more time to heal—will help close that gap.

If you think you need extra help, especially if you have a diastasis larger than three fingers width or if it gets worse, I recommend good, hands-on manual **physical therapy treatment.** That, **along with specific exercises and education on how to prevent increasing abdominal pressure during daily activities,** can bring a faster, more effective recovery.[2] If you do go for **physical therapy treatment,** you can bring this book along and share the **Baby Bod® Exercise Program.** Your therapist will make sure you are doing the exercises correctly, by using good form and the right breathing techniques.

Most doctors and midwives do not realize that physical therapy treatment can help prevent further separation and expedite the closure of the gap between these muscles. So don't wait for your healthcare practitioner to offer a referral; you'll have to take the initiative yourself.

Only in rare cases will surgery be necessary to correct this condition. Even then, physical therapy and exercise are a very important part of the recovery process.

Just don't ignore it. As I said above, women who have diastasis recti are more likely to develop lower back pain, incontinence, and pelvic organ prolapse, conditions you definitely want to stop in their tracks. [2, 3, 4, 5, 6]

Incontinence, yes, we are going there![7, 8, 9, 10]

Did you know that leaking urine is not normal? Not even a few little drops?

In pregnant and postpartum women, **it's common—but not normal**—to leak urine. Fortunately, it is often curable. If you think you have a problem leaking urine, please read the questions in the worksheet below this section and then record your findings on your worksheet. If you do consult with a healthcare professional about leaking urine, bring this chart with you.

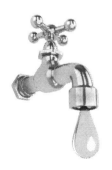

You can more/Shutterstock.com

WORKSHEET

Incontinence Questions: What Are You Experiencing?	No?	Yes?
1. Do you leak pee when you cough, sneeze, run or pick up a grocery package?		
2. Can you hold your urine for 2 ½ hours?		
3. Are you able to urinate with an uninterrupted flow? Or does your flow stop and go?		
4. Do you find yourself making several toilet stops per day, "just in case" you need to go later? Or do you think you have a "tiny bladder"?		
5. Do you always make it to the bathroom on time?		
6. Do you feel any pain or discomfort, like burning, when you pee?		
7. Do you find you have to return to use the toilet moments after you thought you had finished urinating?		
8. Do you need to use pads to prevent urine "spillage" onto your clothing? If so, how many pads per day?		

Use your worksheet.

What can you do to resolve this problem? First, *call or make an appointment with your doctor or midwife and ask them to do a test to see if you have a bladder infection.* If you don't have an infection, follow the advice I give below and try to progress with the **Baby Bod® Program**. If the urine leakage does not resolve after you have tried this exercises program for a month or two, or if your symptoms are getting worse, you may need more intensive one-on-one pelvic physical therapy treatment or even medical treatment from a urologist or urogynecologist. Sometimes, the best treatment comes when your doctor and physical therapist team up. When they collaborate, they can often create a successful treatment program.

In some cases, women report **fecal staining** or **fecal incontinence.** If you fall into that category, record what you are experiencing when it occurs; if it does not go away, report this to your doctor or midwife and seek help. There are some physical therapy treatment options that may help to resolve this uncomfortable problem.

Types of Urinary Leakage

There are two main categories of urinary incontinence: **Stress Incontinence** and **Urge Incontinence**. With Stress Incontinence, women usually leak urine because the pelvic floor muscles became weak as a result of the stress and strains of pregnancy and childbirth or obesity. This is the most common type of urine leakage. It occurs when you exercise, sneeze, laugh or cough. Women with stress incontinence usually get better after a few months of doing the **Baby Bod® Program.**

Contrast that with **Urge Incontinence** (also known as "Overactive Bladder"). The cause of Urge Incontinence can be a little more complex than Stress Incontinence. Women who have Urge Incontinence often complain of an urgent need to urinate frequently and don't always make it to the toilet in time. If you answered yes to questions 3, 4, 5, 6, or 7, you may fall into this category. *The first thing you should do is to call your doctor or midwife and ask for a urine test to make sure you do not have a urinary tract infection.* Women with Urge Incontinence may need more than the exercises offered in this program. My best advice is to try the **Baby Bod® Exercise Program** for a few weeks, and if you do not get better, consider going to a urologist or a urogynecologist for an exam. Also consider going to a women's health physical therapist or physiotherapist for treatments and learn exercises that will help your specific problem.

Eight Causes of Urinary Leakage

1. Pregnancy: The hormonal changes and the pressure exerted on the urinary tract by the extra weight of the growing baby can cause urinary leakage.

**Do You Feel Like You Don't Totally Empty
Your Bladder When You Pee?**

Some women are unable to fully empty their bladder when they urinate, especially right after childbirth. If you feel that you have to return to the toilet shortly after you just went, try this:

After you finish urinating, stand up and rock your pelvis back and forth a few times and then move your pelvis in circles a few times (like the pelvic rock exercises that you'll find in Chapter Thirteen). Then sit down and try to empty the remaining urine in your bladder. Remember: whatever you do, fight the temptation to "push" your urine out when you pee.

Tip: This is usually temporary and resolves shortly after childbirth. The **Baby Bod® Program** can be helpful in preventing this from becoming a lingering problem after childbirth.

2. Muscle Weakness: Many women have weaker pelvic floor muscles from the strain of carrying around excess weight for nine months and the trauma caused by childbirth.

Tip: The exercises in the **Baby Bod® Program** should help resolve urine leakage that is caused by muscle weakness.

3. Urine Blockage: Did you answer yes to question #3 or #7?

Do you find that your urine starts and stops and starts up again? If your stream is interrupted, it could mean that the muscles in your pelvic floor are in spasm.

Tip: Try to do more of the lower tummy breathing and the rib expander breathing exercises you will learn in Chapter Twelve for 10 minutes a few times per day.

Do you find you have to return to use the toilet moments after you thought you had finished urinating? This can be caused by one of the pelvic organs preventing or blocking the flow of urine. If you recently gave birth and you don't have a urinary tract infection, this may just be temporary; it will go away when your uterus shrinks back down to normal size. If it continues, however, it may indicate that you have pelvic organ prolapse, which also may be temporary and may go away once your "pregnancy hormones" balance out again. (See below for more information on this condition.)

Tip: If you do experience this, try emptying your bladder, then stand up and do a few of the pelvic rock exercises described in Chapter Fourteen and then sit down again and see if you can empty more urine. (As tempted as you may be, don't try to force the urine out by pushing!) You may want to consider seeking professional help to evaluate why this is happening to you.

4. Learned Behavior: Because women learn to go to the toilet several more times per day during pregnancy, they can become "trained" to continue to urinate "just in case" they may need to go later on in the day. This is something women become accustomed to doing during pregnancy and continue to do after childbirth even though their bodies are able to hold larger amounts of urine.

Tip: If you do this, try to change this behavior by gradually spreading out the time between toilet trips. You might start by waiting 5 to 10 minutes to urinate after you feel the urge. During that time, do the lower tummy breathing exercises I will teach you in Chapter Fourteen. Then CALMLY walk—don't run—to the toilet to urinate. If you rush to the toilet, you can set off a chain reaction in the body that will virtually guarantee that you will have an accident. This will allow your body to relearn how to hold more urine. Once you are able to wait an extra 5 to 10 minutes, gradually try to extend that time to two hours.

5. Toileting habits: The way you sit can make a difference.

Tip: Read below about the best posture to use when you use the toilet.

Tip: Most moms I know are always in a rush. When you urinate, *don't push your urine out*; your bladder works best when you relax and let the urine come out naturally.

6. Constipation: This is a common problem in both pregnant and postpartum women. It can cause excess strain on the pelvic floor muscles and lead to weakness and leakage.

Tip: To prevent it, make sure you eat enough fiber, stay well hydrated, and get enough exercise.

Tip: Try doing the Constipation Self-Massage I will teach you in the next two chapters. (Please choose the one relevant to the kind of birth you had, whether vaginal or C-section.)

Tip: Read the section below on how use "better toilet posture" to improve your ability to pass a bowel movement.

Tip: If these simple tips do not work, know that there are some pelvic physical therapists and physiotherapists with a lot of experience in treating and resolving constipation. Don't be too embarrassed to seek help.

7. Bladder Irritants: Certain beverages and foods can irritate the bladder wall and can lead to urinary leakage.

Tip: Sometimes, you can end urinary incontinence by keeping yourself well hydrated—the fluids dilute the substances that might otherwise irritate the bladder. *How much water should you drink per day?* It is important not to over-hydrate by drinking too much; but do drink enough to quench your thirst.

Tip: Try avoiding certain foods and drinks that irritate the

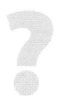

Did You Know?

Diet is more often found to be the cause of urinary leakage than a full bladder. For more information on this, please check out the Interstitial Cystitis Association at http://www.ichelp.org.

bladder. Figuring out what to avoid may take a little trial and error; what's fine for someone else might irritate you. Here are some potential irritants. Try cutting them all out for a time, maybe a week or two, and then introduce them back into your diet one by one. Wait for two days each time you add something back into your diet to see which ones affect you:

+ Foods and beverages that contain artificial ingredients
+ Carbonated drinks
+ Caffeine and chocolate
+ Alcohol
+ Acidic juices such as orange and cranberry
+ Fruits high in acid, like strawberries, pineapples, grapefruits and tomatoes
+ Spicy foods

Summary of Things to Do for Urinary Incontinence:

1. **Follow the Baby Bod® Exercise Program.**
2. Improve toilet habits. (Review the "Healthy Toileting Habits" section below.)
3. Stop "just in case" peeing behavior and try to extend the time in-between "toilet stops."
4. Address constipation issues.
5. Reduce bladder irritants.
6. Reduce strain on the pelvic floor by doing a pelvic floor muscle contraction (which I will teach you later in the book) prior to coughing and sneezing. Also, if you are standing when you sneeze or cough, try lifting one leg prior to sneezing and coughing.
7. If your urine leakage does not improve, seek the help of a health professional.

Healthy Toileting Habits[11, 9]

Before toilets were invented, we all had to squat. Believe it or not, our internal organs were designed to eliminate waste in a squatting position and actually work more efficiently in this position. Squatting can make defecation easier and reduce the need to strain.[11] Modern toilets, which were invented for the safe disposal of bodily wastes, hinder this. *Our bodies were not designed to eliminate stool in the upright-seated position.*

Fortunately, there are simple ways to remedy this without giving up the comfort and privacy of the toilet. I will explain what they are below. First, however, let me explain why they're worth considering. Using a better position to sit on the toilet can help to reduce the risk of developing hemorrhoids. It can also create less stress on the connective tissue inside the pelvis and the pelvic floor and abdominal muscles. **Straining increases the pressure in the abdomen**, and by this point in the book, I hope you have read enough to know that increased intra-abdominal pressure can cause damage to the connective tissue and muscles in the pelvis and abdomen. Increased abdominal pressure can also cause the veins in your anus to swell and develop into hemorrhoids. If you reduce the need to strain by using "healthy toileting habits," you reduce the pressure in the abdomen and prevent damaging your pelvic floor and abdomen and also prevent hemorrhoids.

Here is the best way to empty your bowels:

To Pass a Bowel Movement:

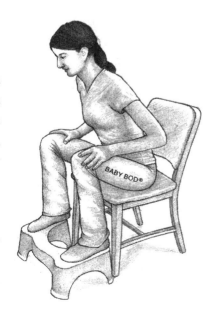

+ Sit with your feet apart. Rest them on a stool that is specifically made for this purpose so that your knees are higher than your hips. In doing research for this book I found the **Squatty Potty**® stool is well designed and an affordable solution. (You can find Squatty Potty® on the Internet and in some retail stores.)
+ Relax your stomach muscles.
+ Lean forward and place your hands on your thighs.
+ Instead of straining to pass the bowel movement, try gently exhaling and saying "mmmmmmm."
+ Do not remain on the toilet for more than 5 to 10 minutes at a time.

Note: Some women find it helpful to use a hand to support the perineum while defecating, especially right after childbirth. (If you are not sure where your perineum is, please refer to the pelvic floor section in Chapter Four). To try this, place a flat hand on your perineum, with your fingers pointing towards your anus and ending just before the anus. As you defecate, use your hand to support this area by gently pushing upwards to make it easier to pass a stool.

When nature calls, do not remain on the toilet for more than 5 to 10 minutes at a time. It is not the best time to catch up on Facebook posts or reading your favorite gossip magazine.

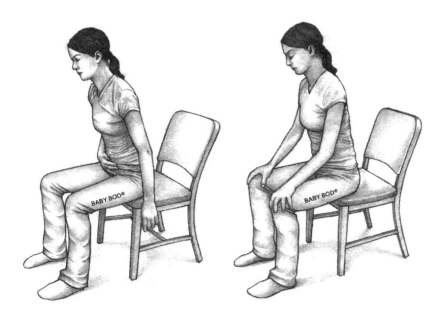

Here is the best way to empty your bladder:

To Urinate:
+ First, sit towards the front of the toilet seat with your feet apart and touching the floor. (If you have a stool, push it to the side and place your feet on the floor.)
+ Use one hand to feel your lower tummy muscles relax.
+ Then lean forward a bit and rest your hands or forearms on your thighs.
+ *Allow your urine to empty without pushing it out.*

Note: It is important to sit on the seat when urinating. ***Don't hover above the seat*** because that position will tighten up your pelvic floor muscles. The opposite has to happen; the pelvic floor muscles need to relax so you can empty your bladder. So try to sit whenever possible, even if you are using a toilet outside of your home. (Use the paper seat liner or toilet paper to line the toilet seat if you are concerned about hygiene.)

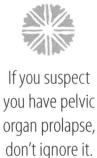

If you suspect
you have pelvic
organ prolapse,
don't ignore it.

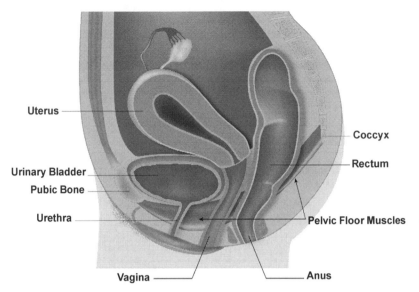

Uterus

Coccyx

Rectum

Urinary Bladder

Pubic Bone

Urethra

Pelvic Floor Muscles

Vagina

Anus

PELVIC ORGAN PROLAPSE

I discussed pelvic organ prolapse (or POP) earlier. The degree of slippage varies. As you saw in the story I told you about my client, Megan, the amount an organ slips down can be made worse by certain activities, especially activities that can increase the pressure inside your abdomen, such as heavy lifting, sit-up exercises, and straining when you pass a bowel movement. POP can interfere with normal bowel and bladder functioning. It can also lead to several complications such as incontinence, pelvic and back pain and sexual dysfunctions.

How do I know if I have Pelvic Organ Prolapse?

If you have reason to believe you might have pelvic organ prolapse, here are questions I would like you to ask yourself:

WORKSHEET

Pelvic Organ Prolapse Questions	✓ Yes?
Do you feel as if there's "something" in your vagina?	
Do you feel as if something seems to be coming out of or pushing down on your pelvic floor every time you cough, sneeze, or jump?	
Can you feel something coming out of your vagina, especially after passing a bowel movement?	
When you urinate, are you able to fully empty your bladder?	
Do you leak urine, or have a constant "dribble" of urine leaking from your bladder?	
Do you have a constant urge to urinate?	
Do you have to return to the toilet to empty your bladder shortly after you urinate?	
Are you able to fully empty your bowels at one time, or do you need to return frequently to finish making a bowel movement?	

Please record and date your answers on the worksheet. This way you'll remember important details when you talk with your physician, midwife, pelvic physical therapist or woman's health physiotherapist.

If you said YES to some of the questions above, it could indicate that you have a prolapse of one or more of your pelvic organs. It *may be temporary* if you recently gave birth. If you suspect you have pelvic organ prolapse, *don't* ignore it. Get the condition evaluated by a healthcare professional. He or she can tell you whether the prolapse is mild, moderate, or severe and what your treatment options are. Severe cases may require surgery.

Studies have shown that physical therapy treatment can reduce or resolve POP for some women. [6, 12, 13] The evidence so far has shown that mild cases can be resolved with pelvic physical therapy treatment and more severe cases can be reduced. That means that physical therapy can PREVENT SURGERY.

Note: At the time this book went to press, one of the most recent studies on surgery for pelvic organ prolapse showed that one third of these surgeries fail within seven years. [14] In other words, the prolapse returns. So it's much smarter to resolve it if you can, rather than rely on surgery, because the results may not be permanent.

Self-Care for Pelvic Organ Prolapse

As with diastasis recti, the first thing you want to do is **prevent pelvic organ prolapse from getting worse** by protecting your abdomen and pelvic floor, especially when your body is still under the influence of the lingering effect of the "pregnancy hormones." This can last three months after childbirth, or, if you are breastfeeding, the entire time you nurse your child plus three months after you wean your child. During this time, you'll want to follow the same advice I just gave regarding diastasis recti. (Since you have already read that, let me just summarize it on the next page.)

Things to Avoid When You Have Pelvic Organ Prolapse:

1. **Avoid strenuous activities or exercises that place strain on the abdomen or pelvic floor or increases the pressure inside your abdomen.** Increased abdominal pressure will push the organs downwards and you will risk making the POP worse. If you do have to engage in an activity that requires exertion, make sure to EXHALE as you perform the activity.

2. **Avoid "Jackknife behavior,"** such as getting up from bed or up from the floor as if you are doing a sit-up.

3. **Avoid stiff or tight elastic abdominal binders.** The compression from an abdominal binder causes a downward force that can cause the pelvic organs to descend further and could make your condition worse.

4. **Do what you can to prevent constipation.** Remember that straining increases the pressure in your abdomen and this can cause

the pelvic organs to move further down towards your pelvic floor.

Things to Do: Caring for Pelvic Organ Prolapse

1. Consider wearing a **Pelvic Floor Support Belt,** especially when you exercise or stand for long periods of time. (See Chapters Eight and Nine to find out more information.)

2. If you have moderate to severe prolapse, consider discussing using a pessary with your health care provider. A **pessary** is a medical device that is inserted into the vagina to help add additional support to the pelvic organs and needs to be fitted by the appropriate healthcare provider.

3. Wear a pair of **long-waisted shorts with medical grade graduated compression** during the day for at least a few months after childbirth. DO NOT wear tight shape-wear as a substitute. If you do not want to wear a compression garment, you may want to try using the Baby Bod® Abdominal Wrap. You can read more about compression garments and the wrap in Chapters Eight and Nine.

4. Try wearing a **Pelvic/SI Belt** and/or a **Pelvic Floor Support Belt** to add a little more support. (See whether the Pelvic/SI Belt works best for you when you look at the directions for the Straight Leg Raise Test in Chapter Five.) (You can wear both belts at the same time.)

5. Use **good body mechanics** to prevent excess pressure on your pelvic floor and internal organs. See "Get Your **Baby Bod**® On All Day Long" in Chapter Seventeen.

6. Try doing the **Abdominal and Pelvic Floor Massages** that you will find in the next two chapters on self-care. (Again, there is a chapter for women who had a vaginal birth and another one for women who had a C-section. Please read the chapter that pertains to you.)

7. **Exhale** when you exert yourself to prevent pressure from building up inside your abdomen. Make sure the amount you exhale matches the level of activity. Try to not to hold your breath when lifting, pushing and pulling.

8. Use **good bladder and bowel habits,** which I have described above.

9. Prevent **constipation** by eating a good diet with plenty of fiber. Drink a lot of water and try doing the **Constipation Self-Massage** that's in the self-care chapters.

10. **Reduce strain on the pelvic floor** by doing a pelvic floor muscle contraction (which I will teach you later in the book) prior to coughing and sneezing. Also, if you are standing when you sneeze or cough, try lifting one leg prior to sneezing and coughing.

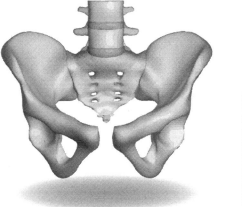

Oscar Moncho/Shutterstock.com

11. Do the **Baby Bod® exercises** provided for you in this book. If you've just had your baby, you're in a particularly good position to halt the progression of prolapse because you have **Baby Bod®** in your hands now. **Baby Bod®** can help to resolve milder cases of prolapse or prevent it from getting worse. Just give it a little time to work. It will shore up your pelvic floor and core muscles, which will

tighten up the ligaments that support pelvic organs. Tightening the ligaments can prevent the downward migration of your pelvic organs.

Try these tips for a couple of weeks and re-assess the situation. If you find it getting worse, it could be that you are doing the exercises wrong or lifting (the baby, the groceries, etc.) the wrong way. Either way, it is important for you to seek professional help. You may need to consider consulting a doctor and a women's health physical therapist or physiotherapist for treatment.

Pubic Symphysis Dysfunction [7, 8]

In the chapter on anatomy, I made mention of this condition. Let me give you a recap here: As you recall, the pubic symphysis joint separates the front of the pelvis into right and left sides. It becomes even more flexible under the influence of the "pregnancy hormones." If the joint moves too much, which is more likely to happen toward the last trimester of pregnancy, it can cause excess movement in the front of the pelvis and pain in the groin or in the pubic symphysis joint. Postpartum women can also develop pain in this area, especially after a vaginal birth. In severe cases the pelvis can separate in this area.

This is one of the most common misdiagnosed problems I see in my clinic.

This is one of the most common misdiagnosed problems I see in my clinic. Since women who have pubic symphysis dysfunction complain of pain in the in the groin area, especially when they're walking, standing and climbing stairs, some doctors and midwives misdiagnose their problem as *hip pain*. Some women are given a cane or walker to use to take weight off their "hips" and to make it easier to get around. Many women who come into my office for treatment need to walk sideways to decrease the pain.

Pubic Symphysis ◆ A Case Story

I recently treated a woman, Karen, who told me she had pain in the front of her pelvis and groin prior to delivering her baby. Her doctor told her it was coming from her hip and she should consider using a cane when walking. After childbirth, she was unable to get up off the delivery table without severe pain and could not put any weight on her legs when she was told to stand up. The doctor said that she had probably strained her hip during delivery and that it would get better on its own. Karen was sent home with a walker and told to use it until the pain went away. Luckily, she found my office on the Internet and called me and asked if I thought I would be able to help her. I assured her over the phone that she most likely had a common problem related to her pregnancy called pubic symphysis dysfunction and that it was probably made worse from the trauma of childbirth.

When she came in to see me, she told me that she had been living with severe pain since she had delivered her baby ten days earlier. I evaluated her condition, then I addressed the torsion in her pelvis with manual physical therapy and also gave her a Pelvic/ SI Belt to wear.

After that first session, Karen was able to leave the walker behind and walk out of my office unassisted. She came in for two more visits to learn a few of the **Baby Bod® exercises** and also to learn how to prevent straining her pelvis while it healed. By the time she was three weeks postpartum, she was pain-free and a happy mom. She was able to progress with the program on her own at home after that.

How to Care for Pubic Symphysis Dysfunction: Things to Avoid

Care should be taken during the last two trimesters of pregnancy, during childbirth, and after delivery to prevent developing pubic symphysis dysfunction. Here are some things to avoid during the last two trimesters and for at least a month or two after childbirth:

- **Avoid one-legged activities** that can put a strain on the pelvis, such as pushing a heavy box with one leg, swinging your leg to hop on a bicycle, or climbing a ladder. (This also includes avoiding certain yoga poses that require you to stand on one leg, such as the Tree and the Warrior Pose, because they put a lot of torsional force on the pubic symphysis).

+ Consider **safer labor positions** that will decrease straining the pubic symphysis during delivery, such as side-lying, or positioning yourself on your hands and knees, or modified squat and standing positions. The typical birthing position used in hospitals, lying on your back, creates the most amount of strain in the pubic symphysis area. It can cause this problem or make it worse.

What to Do If You Have Pubic Symphysis Dysfunction

+ **Manual physical therapy** can address the torsion on your pelvis and help you get immediate relief. The right types of exercises will help prevent it from reoccurring during the remainder of your pregnancy and after delivery.

+ Try using a **Pelvic/SI Belt** if you are postpartum. Pregnant women can try using a pregnancy support belt.

+ Use **good body mechanics** in all your daily activities. See the "Get Your **Baby Bod**® on All Day Long" and self-care chapters. Pay special attention to the instructions on how to use a log roll to move around in bed, and how to get up from a chair or bed.

+ **Exhale** when exerting yourself.

+ Try to **sleep with a pillow between your legs** to decrease straining the pelvis.

If you are in pain, consider using a **cane** when walking around to add additional support to the pelvis. (Use the cane on the side opposite to your more painful side.) In severe cases, use a walker to take the pressure off the pubic symphysis.

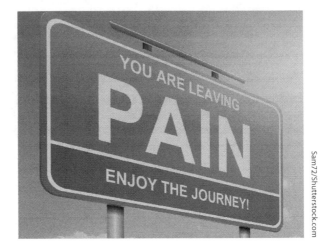

Sam72/Shutterstock.com

Be proactive and see a physical therapist for pain relief. Why live with pain?

POST-PREGNANCY PAIN

It's normal to feel sore for a week or so after giving birth. In the ideal world, you'd see a pelvic physical therapist for a postpartum check-up soon after you give birth and then begin the **Baby Bod® Preliminary Exercises.** If you do that, you should notice the pain diminishing quickly. But if you do not see a physical therapist for a postpartum check-up and you still have the same consistent pain in your back or pelvis beyond a week or two after giving birth, you need help. Make sure to report this to your doctor or midwife and then consider making an appointment with a women's health physical therapist for an evaluation. Pain is a signal that something's wrong. Don't ignore the signal.

It's best to nip problems like this in the bud, before they get worse. Pain that lasts for more than three months (it does not have to be consistently hurting you 24/7) is considered chronic pain. Did you know that *chronic pain* is much harder to resolve than acute pain? So strike when the iron is hot and get the pain relief you deserve early on.

If you are in pain, it would be a good idea to note here what you're experiencing and/or what activity caused it and when. This way you'll have the details handy when you consult a healthcare professional. Please record and date your observations on your worksheet in this section.

W O R K S H E E T

Pain After Childbirth	Yes? Give a Brief Description	No
On a Scale of 1 to 10, with 10 being the worst, how would you rate your pain?		
What makes the pain worse?		
What makes the pain better?		
Is it worse in the morning, afternoon or evening?		
Does the pain interfere with sleeping?		
Do you feel it when you're getting up from sitting down?		
Or when you're sitting?		
Or when you're walking?		
Or going up a set of stairs?		
Or when you are passing a bowel movement or urinating?		
Is it interfering with your life, with your normal everyday activities?		
How much can you walk without pain?		
What activity causes the most pain?		
Does the pain prevent you from exercising?		

If you simply can't find any resting position that feels good or is NOT painful, or if you find the pain getting worse even though you're doing the **Baby Bod® Program**, stop the program and get proper treatment for your pain first. You can resume later.

Please don't assume that pain is something you have to live with—it *isn't*.[D] **Pain may be common among women right after childbirth, but if it lingers for more than a week or so, it's not normal.** Don't be swayed by anyone who might tell you the pain will go away on its own, whether that's your neighbor, a family member or healthcare professional. Instead, be proactive and see a physical therapist for pain relief. Why live with pain? I'm saying this because in my practice I've seen too many women who endured pain after delivery and didn't even think of mentioning it to their doctors or midwives until their six-week checkup.

I also see new mothers who finally come in for an evaluation after they return to work when they are anywhere from three to six months postpartum; they finally realize that in order to keep up with their hectic lifestyle as a working mom, they better get help. They suffered needlessly, because a lot of these problems could be resolved after a few physical therapy visits.

Finally, don't let an overwhelming schedule dissuade you from making that appointment. You'll be surprised at what can be accomplished in just a few visits. If your issues can't be resolved in a visit or two, you can always schedule follow-up visits down the road when your schedule is less packed.

Tips to Relieve Pelvic Pain

In the self-care chapters that come next, I'll provide you with several different tips on how to relieve pain right after delivery. I will also go over specific self-massages you can use to help in your recovery. Some of these can help relieve muscle spasms and scar tissue pain weeks or months after childbirth. Here are other ways to help relieve pain:

[D] Note: This advice is for pregnant women also. I have seen pregnant women endure back pain for many months longer than they should have because when they mentioned it to their healthcare professional they were told that it was normal to feel aches and pains during pregnancy and they would eventually go away on their own. And since they usually have monthly visits with their healthcare professional, it could take a few months of continued complaints before they are told to go to a physical therapist for treatment.

- Try to do the **breathing exercises** (Lower Abdominal Breathing and Rib Expanders) in Chapter Twelve with two or three pillows under your buttocks and extend the time you do them to 10 minutes each at least one to two times a day. It is a nice way to relax before falling asleep. You can also do it in the side-lying position while nursing or feeding your baby. Try doing a few minutes of Lower Tummy Breathing Exercises just before engaging in intercourse; this can help decrease your discomfort during sex.

- Try taking a warm bath to relax your pelvic floor muscles.

- Try sitting on a donut-shaped pillow to relieve pressure on the pelvic floor area.

- Try doing some of the warm up exercises, especially the pelvic rocks mentioned in Chapter Fourteen, to loosen up tight muscles.

- Read the advice on good toileting habits in this chapter and learn the most efficient way to urinate and defecate. Many women have a tendency to "push" their urine out, and that could cause the muscles in your pelvic floor to tighten and possibly go into spasm.

- Try doing the **Constipation Self-Massage** found in the self-care chapters Eight and Nine, and use the good toileting postures mentioned earlier in this chapter. Constipation can cause you to develop muscle spasms if you use a lot of force to push a bowel movement out.

- Try doing the **Abdominal** and **Pelvic Floor Massages** that are mentioned in the self-care chapters Eight and Nine. Make sure to use some lubrication if you have a lot of dryness in your vagina.

+ You can start the **Baby Bod® Program**, but make sure to use only gentle contractions when you do the *Pelvic-Core Starter* exercise.

Try following these steps for a few weeks and see if it helps. If you feel like your symptoms are getting worse, report it to your doctor or midwife and consider going for physical therapy treatment. Don't think that you need to be "Superwoman" and do this all on your own. There are capable professionals who are more than willing to help you restore your body to full function again!

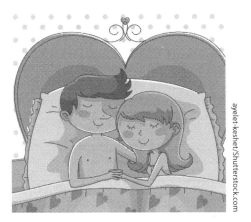

ayelet-keshet/Shutterstock.com

Painful Sex after Baby

Do you experience pain during sex? Perhaps you haven't questioned whether this is "normal" because you've talked this over with some of your girlfriends and found out they've experienced it, too. But just because something is common, it doesn't make it "normal."

Initially, most women feel some discomfort when they try to "get back in the saddle" again and resume sexual intercourse after childbirth. Here's what you can do to eliminate or reduce the pain:

+ First, use some of the **pain relief tips** I mentioned above.

+ Prior to having intercourse, try to take a warm bath to relax.

+ After you've toweled off, try using a vaginal lubricant prior to having sex. Make sure to buy one that does not have glycerin in it, because glycerin can dry out the skin and cause vaginal dryness, rather than helping it.

+ You also need to have a frank discussion with your partner about the pain you're feeling. Let your partner know that right now—for the time being—he or she can help reduce the pain by providing lots of foreplay before penetration, and also by limiting the depth and duration of the penetration. Remind your partner that this is temporary, just until you heal.

+ One of the guidelines I give women is **do not engage in intercourse if it is painful.** Wait until you can have intercourse, even modified intercourse, without pain.

These tips should help. There are several reasons why you may experience pain during sex. If the pain persists for a few months after you deliver your baby, it is NOT NORMAL. That's an indication you need professional care. If the pain does not go away, I would like to make you aware that women's health physical therapists and physiotherapists are trained to help you regain your sex life again by using several different treatment methods to relieve the pain.

Get right on any small problems before they become large problems.

* * *

I hope the advice I have given you in this chapter has been helpful. It puts the power back in your hands so you can get right on any small problems before they become large problems. In the next chapters, we'll look at self-care immediately after giving birth. If you had a vaginal birth, please turn to the next chapter. If you had a C-section, please skip the next chapter and turn to Chapter Nine. And if it's been months or years since you gave birth, you can skip most of the information in both chapters, but do take a look at the self-massages in the chapter that pertains to you and try them out.

[1] Boissonnault JS, Blaschak MJ. Incidence of Diastasis Recti Abdominis During the Childbearing Year. *Phys Ther.* July 1988; 68(7):1082-1086. http://ptjournal.apta.org/content/68/7/1082

[2] Parker MA, Millar AL, Dugan SA. Diastasis Rectus Abdominis and Lumbo-Pelvic Pain and Dysfunction-Are They Related? *Journal of Women's Health Physical Therapy.* Spring 2008; 32:1. http://www.meredyparkerpt.com/pdfs/Meredy%20Article.pdf

[3] Spitnagle TM, Leong FC, Van Dillen LR. Prevalence of diastasis rectus abdominis in a urogynecological patient population. *Int Urogynecol J.* 2007 ; 18(3):321-8. doi:10.1007/s00192-006-0143-5

[4] Lo T, Candido G, Janssen P. Diastasis of the recti abdominis in pregnancy: Risk factors and treatment. *Physiother Canada.* 1999; 51(I):32-37,44.

[5] Sheppard S. The Role of Transversus Abdominis in Post Partum Correction of Gross Divarication Recti. *Man Ther.* 1996; 1(4):214-216. doi: 10.1054/math.1996.0272.

[6] Braekken IH, Majida M, Ellström EM, Holme IM, Bo K. Pelvic floor function is independently associated with pelvic organ prolapse. *BJOG.* 2009 Dec; 116(13):1706-14. doi: 10.1111/j.1471-0528.2009.02379.x.

[7] Laycock J, Haslam J. *Therapeutic Management of Incontinence and Pelvic Pain.* London, UK: Springer-Verlag London Limited; 2002.

[8] Stephenson RG, O'Conner LJ. *Obstetric and Gynecologic Care in Physical Therapy 2nd Edition.* Thorofare,NJ: SLACK Incorporated; 2000.

[9] Sapsford R, Bullock-Saxton J, Markwell S. *Women's Health: A Textbook for Physiotherapists.* Oval Road, London, UK::WB Saunders Company Ltd; 1998.

[10] Carriere B, Feldt CM. *The Pelvic Floor.* Rudigerstrasse, Stuttgart, Germany: Georg Thieme Verlag; 2006.

[11] Sakakibara R, Tsunoyama K, Hosoi H, et al. Influence of Body Position on Defecation in Humans. *LUTS: Lower Urinary Tract Symptoms.* 11 Jan 2010; 2(1):16-21. doi: 10.1111/j.1757-5672.2009.00057.x.

[12] Hagen S, Stark D. Conservative prevention and management of pelvic organ prolapse in women. *Cochrane Database Syst Rev.* 2011 Dec 7; (12):CD003882. doi: 10.1002/14651858. CD003882.pub4.

[13] Hagen S, Stark D, Glazener C, et al. Individualised pelvic floor muscle training in women with organ prolapse (Poppy): a multicenter randomized controlled trial. *The Lancet.* 1 March 2014; 383(9919):796-806. doi:10.1016/S0140-6736(13)61977-7.

[14] Nygaard I, Brubaker L, Zyczynski HM, et al. Long-term outcomes following abdominal sacrocolpopexy for pelvic organ prolapse. JAMA. 2013 May 15; 309(19):2016-24. doi: 10.1001/*JAMA*.2013.4919.

Self-Care After a Vaginal Birth

The time right after delivery is very exciting; the flood of endorphins may keep you going for a week or so. But if you are anything like me, well, I finally hit the wall on postpartum day ten. Rather than feeling fabulous, I woke up feeling like a Mack truck hit me sometime in the night. The sleep deprivation started to get the better of me and I had aches and pains in body parts I didn't even know I had.

Sound familiar? If this is your first child, it can be very disconcerting. After enduring so many uncomfortable changes during pregnancy, you're looking forward to getting your body back to normal. This doesn't happen instantly, something you know full well if this isn't your first baby. If it is, I hope you read the earlier chapters that explain *why*. You do have to be patient as Nature takes its course, but there are *smart* ways to help Nature along. Knowing *WHAT to do WHEN* and *WHAT NOT to do* can make a big difference. In this chapter, I'll cover basic self-care measures which—in addition to the **Baby Bod® exercises**—will put your recovery into high gear.

Your Individual Plan

The advice below is for all moms who had or plan to have a vaginal delivery. (If you had a C-section delivery, please skip this chapter and read the next chapter).

+ Ideally, you'll have this book in hand when you are *pregnant*, so you can make use of all the good advice in this chapter and start the program before you give birth. You will find some of the advice handy to use right after you deliver your baby.

Basic self-care measures will put your recovery into high gear.

+ If you are starting this program *right after delivery*, you are right on target.

+ If you are starting this program *a few weeks after childbirth*, please do the self-tests and self-massages included in this chapter. Then start the *Preliminary Phase* of exercises for at least one week and until you have your six-week checkup.

+ If you are starting this program after your six-week checkup (even months or years after you've last given birth), please do at least a week of the **Baby Bod® Preliminary Phase Exercises**, along with the self-tests and massages below, before progressing to the more challenging strengthening exercises in the second phase of **Baby Bod®**.

Tip # 1: Don't Be in a Rush to Resume Your Normal Routine

As I said in Chapter Five, it takes—on average—about six weeks to complete just the *first stage* of soft tissue (connective tissue) healing after delivery. It will take at least *another six to eight weeks* for your ligaments and connective tissue to return to "normal" if you are not breastfeeding. (That is a total of THREE months after childbirth.) If you are breastfeeding, however, it can take up to *three months after you stop nursing* for your connective tissue to regain the ability to support your body like it did before you got pregnant. Also, your abdominal and pelvic floor muscles need time to heal. If you don't give them time—and you strain them during this period—recovery will take that much longer.

So don't even think about jumping back into your regular routine right away! *Embrace a gradual recovery.* To tell you the truth, *I personally consider the recovery from childbirth equivalent to recovering from major surgery.* If you can put off returning to work for at least three months after you've given birth, do. (More time off from work than that is optimal.)

Tip # 2: Get Help with Taxing Household Tasks

As I said to pregnant women in an earlier chapter, arrange for help with household tasks that are physically taxing, like grocery shopping and house cleaning. Don't be afraid to ask. Have someone else do the heavy lifting when setting up—or re-arranging—the nursery. And imprint this one rule brain: Do not lift or push anything heavier than your newborn baby for the first six weeks after you had your baby.

This includes carrying grocery bags, strollers, laundry baskets and the like. You also want to avoid pushing a vacuum or pushing open heavy doors until you reach the six-week postpartum benchmark. (In Chapter Seventeen, I'll talk more about how to move around safely with as little strain as possible.)

Tip # 3: Carve Out Time to Learn the Baby Bod® Preliminary Phase Exercises

If you are reading this book while you are pregnant, it is best to learn how to do the **Preliminary Phase of Baby Bod®** *now*, to make it easier after you deliver. As I said earlier, these exercises are safe for pregnant women and will benefit you. If you are reading this right after delivery, start the program slowly, and follow each step.

At the risk of repeating myself, I don't advocate *complete* rest after childbirth—except for the select few of you with pregnancy-related disorders or childbirth complications where complete rest is appropriate. This is the perfect time to start the **Baby Bod® Preliminary Phase Exercises** because your body needs to move to keep the blood circulating, which is an important part of the healing process. If you are too sedentary, it interrupts the normal flow of blood to the tissues, which can delay healing and make you feel stiff and tired.

You'll find these exercises in Chapters Eleven to Fourteen. The window of time between the day after you give birth and your postpartum checkup is the perfect time to do them. Getting an early start will help build a solid foundation for the more progressive exercises that follow.

Doing **Baby Bod®** benefits you in two ways: In terms of time, you get a jump-start because you start six weeks earlier than most other moms. And in terms of results, your muscles will be "awake

Do not lift or push anything heavier than your newborn baby for the first 6 weeks after you had your baby.

and ready" after those initial six weeks to get great results from the more progressive strengthening exercises that follow, unlike those moms who didn't do this program and who haven't yet recovered full function in their core muscles.

DAY-BY-DAY HEALING GUIDE

If you've had a normal vaginal birth, you can follow the advice below without reservation.[A] **If you've had a Grade 3 or 4 tear**, however (and by that I mean either a large partial or total tear in the perineum, vagina and or anal sphincter—-be sure to ask your doctor or midwife if you fall into this category), you may need to delay starting some parts of the **Preliminary Phase Exercises** during the first six postpartum weeks. (Please read the sidebar, "Perineal and Vaginal Tears," later on in this chapter. Also be sure to read my specific advice, which is in boldface for those of you with a Grade 3 or 4 tear. You can also look at the chart below for clarification if you need it.)

If you skipped the chapter for pregnant women because you already had your baby, here are some things I mentioned that you might want to keep handy in the early days after childbirth:

- At least 2 dozen **non-latex gloves**. (You'll pack these with ice and use them for pain relief.)
- Microwavable **moist heating pads**. These will be handy to relieve neck and lower back pain. Use the pads for 15 minutes at a time.
- Special items that can help support your body, such as the **Baby Bod® Abdominal Wrap, medical grade compression shorts** with a **long-waist**, a **pelvic/SI Belt** and possibly a **Pelvic Floor Support Belt**. I'll talk about these in a bit.
- **A donut-shaped pillow to sit on.**
- **Two tennis balls inside a tube sock** to be used to roll over sore muscles.
- **Sitz bath**
- **Peri bottle**

[A] If you've had a Cesarean section, please turn to the next chapter.

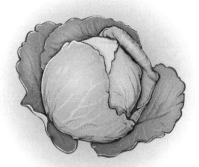

Codrut Crososchi/Shutterstock.com

Do Cabbage Leaves Relieve Pain? Or Is That a Myth?

Many new mothers report that making a compress of fresh cabbage leaves and placing it on their breasts helps relieve the pain of engorgement. I never tried this myself, but you might want to give it a go.

A study done by the Cochrane Pregnancy and Childbirth Group showed that cabbage leaves can help to relieve the discomfort and pain many women experience during the engorgement phase, although researchers are not absolutely sure why. [1] Mothers who do this boil the cabbage, then let it cool down to room temperature or chill it. Then they crush it so that the veins on the leaves are broken. They place a few crushed leaves on the breast for about twenty minutes and apply the compress three to four times a day during the engorgement phase. [2]

This is probably safe to try unless you are allergic to sulfa drugs because the cabbage leaves contain sulfa. So if you have a sulfa drug allergy, steer clear. (If you are not sure whether you can tolerate sulfa, try doing a "skin patch test" by putting a piece of boiled cabbage on your forearm for twenty-four hours first.)

SELF-CARE CHART

Here's a chart you can start using right after you deliver your child and continue to use for a couple of months.

Note: The garments listed in the chart below are *suggestions* to help support your body during the healing phase. You may find them helpful for months and even years after childbirth. Most moms pick and choose which supportive garments work best for them. I'll talk more about these below.

HEALING TIMELINE * * *	Vaginal Delivery	Grade 3 or 4 Tear or Episiotomy
What to Do...	**When to Start...**	**When to Start...**
Ice-packed gloves on pelvic floor	Right after delivery	Right after delivery
Sitz bath	24 hours after delivery	Get medical clearance first
Walk	6 to 8 hours after delivery. (Get medical clearance first.)	6 to 8 hours after delivery. (Get medical clearance first.)
Preliminary Phase Exercises (you'll find these in Chapters 11-14).	24-48 hours after delivery	24-48 hours after delivery. (No *Pelvic-Core Starter* until 6 weeks.)
Baby Bod® Abdominal Wrap – wear 10 to 12 hours a day, especially when you are up and about. Remove or loosen it when you are sitting down.	24 hours after delivery	24 hours after delivery
Long-waisted medical-grade compression shorts 10–12 hours per day	24 hours after delivery	24 hours after delivery
Pelvic/SI Belt for support, if it helps, when you're up and about. (In Chapter 5, you'll find a quick self-test, the *Straight Leg Raise–Core Stability Test*, which will help you determine if you're a candidate for the SI Belt.)	24-48 hours	24-48 hours, but wait until after your six-week checkup before performing the Straight Leg Raise Test.
Pelvic Floor Support Belt. When necessary, wear when you are up and about for 10 to 12 hours.	24 hours after delivery	24 hours after delivery (as long as it does not increase pain).

HEALING TIMELINE * * * *(continued)*	Vaginal Delivery	Grade 3 or 4 Tear or Episiotomy
Straight Leg Raise–Core Stability Test (you'll find this in Chapter 5)	48 hours after delivery	6 weeks after delivery. Wait until you have medical clearance to exercise.
Diastasis Recti Test (found in Chapter 7)	48 hours after delivery	6 to 8 weeks after delivery. Wait until you have medical clearance to exercise.
Abdominal Massages (found below): 1. Abdominal Circles 2. Constipation Massage 3. Diastasis Recti Massage 4. Skin Rolling	Start all abdominal massages a few days after delivery, except for Skin Rolling. Start Skin Rolling one month after you start the other abdominal massages.	Start all abdominal massages a few days after delivery, except for Skin Rolling. Start Skin Rolling one month after you start the other abdominal massages.
Pelvic Floor Massages (found below): 1. Perineal Scar Tissue Massage 2. Pelvic Floor Trigger Point Massage	Start 6 weeks after delivery.	Start 6 weeks after delivery.

* * * You can find all of these items in the **Baby Bod® Store** at *www.BabyBodBook.com.* You'll find the site useful as a reference, even if get your garments elsewhere.

IMMEDIATELY AFTER BIRTH – PAIN RELIEF TIPS

Ice Is Nice

One great way to relieve the immediate pain after childbirth is to fill a non-latex glove with ice, wrap it with a thin cloth and apply it to your pelvic floor area. (Do not apply the ice-filled glove directly on your skin without a thin cloth to protect your skin.) Use one of these glove ice packs as much as possible during the first forty-eight hours after birth, whenever you are resting or sitting. Replace the ice glove with a new clean glove and cloth each time. (Using a new glove and cloth will guard against infection.) If you continue to feel pain after the first forty-eight-hour period, use the ice packs several times a day for around fifteen minutes at a time when you're feeding or nursing your baby or resting. Continue this practice until the pain goes away.

I promise you, applying ice really works to control the pain! I had a large episiotomy after my first child and the ice totally eliminated the pain so I didn't need to take any pain medication. I did this after each birth.

Other Helpful Tips to Relive Pain:

Here are other things you can do to *relieve or prevent* aches and pains in your pelvis, back, upper back or neck. *Try:*

1. Using a **sitz bath** 24 hours after delivery to relieve pain in your bottom. It is a plastic bowl that sits on top of your toilet seat; you will usually be given one during your stay in the hospital. Fill it with lukewarm water and sit in it for about 10 to 15 minutes at a time. The water should feel warm, but not so hot that it burns. You may need to refill the water as you sit on it to keep the temperature warm.

2. Sitting on a **donut-shaped pillow**. These come in handy to relieve aches and pains in your perineum and from hemorrhoids.

3. Using a **peri bottle** that is made out of flexible plastic to ease discomfort or stinging when you urinate. Fill the bottle with warm water and squirt it on your bottom as you pee. Then gently pat yourself dry with toilet paper or tissues. Continue to use a peri bottle until the pain or stinging goes away, which could take a few weeks. It is also nice to use to clean the bloody vaginal discharge (lochia) you will be experiencing during the early postpartum days.

4. Using a **microwavable heating pad** to relieve muscle tension in your back or neck one or two times a day for about 15 minutes at a time. You can use the pad when you are feeding your baby; that way you will be doing two good things at once.

5. Slipping two **tennis balls** into an old sock and then tying a

knot in the sock. Use it as a massage tool to roll over sore muscles. (Don't sit on them.)

6. Learning **good toilet posture** to decrease strain on the pelvic floor. (I covered this in Chapter Seven.)

7. **Preventing Constipation**: A lot of new mothers complain of constipation right after childbirth. You may be given a stool softener to take to make it easier to pass a bowel movement or your doctor may prescribe a gentle laxative. Below, I will guide you through a very effective self-massage you can use to help "push things along." Walking and moving around is also helpful in preventing **constipation. Also, make sure to use** good toileting posture. For more information on this, please refer to the section on Healthy Toileting Habits in Chapter Seven.

8. Wearing **compressive garments** and **Pelvic Support Belts**, which may also reduce pain. We will discuss them later in this chapter.

9. Using **good body mechanics** when you move around. Don't be surprised if you experience pain during everyday activities like rolling in bed or getting out of a chair right after you deliver your child. These simple activities can strain your weak abdominal and pelvic floor muscles and even cause pain. This is why postpartum moms need to protect these areas to prevent further damage and help promote healing. To help you do that, I provide instructions a little later on how to move around in bed and how to get out of a bed or chair with the least amount of effort or strain on your body. In Chapters Sixteen and Seventeen, I will give you even more advice on how to protect your body after childbirth.

That said, if you are in pain, DON'T KEEP SILENT. Make sure you discuss this with your doctor, midwife, doula or nurse.

Motion Is Lotion

After you've given birth, REST as much as possible during the first week. That doesn't mean you should stay in bed the whole time. The more you sit around in bed, the more likely you are to develop stiffness and aches and pain. In fact, get out of bed as soon as you have been given medical clearance and **walk.** *Make sure* there is a medical professional there to assist you the first time you try to get out of bed. I am not talking about a brisk walk. Think *gentle stroll.* You can walk around your hospital room or your home several times during the day. These don't have to be power walks. You might feel sore, but the stiffness should go away quickly once you begin moving around. Try for little ten-minute walks twice a day. If you're still at the hospital, you can walk up and down the hallways. And even if you can't do ten minutes, try for a few minutes at a time and build up to ten.

When you return home, remind yourself to move during the day. We physical therapists have a saying: "Motion is lotion." You need to keep your body moving to keep the blood circulating, which keeps your bones and muscles healthy. Movement also increases the healthy fluids in your joints, which will prevent stiffness. When you are sedentary, it interrupts the normal flow of blood to the tissues. That leads to stiffness and feelings of fatigue.

Even small movements can help. When you sit to nurse or feed your baby, or sit at your computer, try to change positions a few times. And when you can't move that much, you can still combat stiffness with small movements like moving your head around to stretch out your neck muscles, rolling your shoulders, or arching and rounding out your back to stretch out your back muscles. In short, move! This will keep you flexible—and energetic.

Moving Around and Sitting Up in Bed:

Here's a sequence you can use to protect your tummy and pelvic floor when you're getting up from bed. It takes a few steps to learn this. The first thing you need to realize is that you want to *roll over* in bed—as I will explain—*instead of lifting your body up as if you are doing a sit-up.* (Another name for this is "jackknife

Movement prevents developing stiffness, aches and pains.

behavior.") If you are lying on your back, for instance, do NOT lift your head and chest off the bed first. Instead, use a *log roll* to roll yourself to the side of the bed before getting up, and then push yourself up sideways. And remember to EXHALE as you move around to prevent building up the kind of internal pressure that will make your belly bulge. (I covered this in detail in the earlier chapter on the core muscles.)

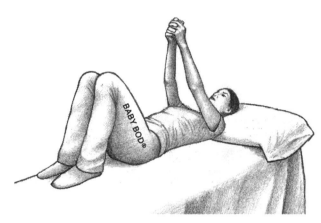

How to Roll Over in Bed (*Log Roll*)

1. Lie on your back and bend your knees. Clasp your fingers together and raise your arms up towards the ceiling.

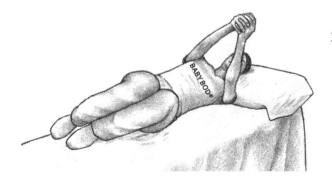

2. *Gently **EXHALE**,* as if you are cleaning your sunglasses. Move your arms and knees at the same time as you slowly roll to one side. (Roll over like a log.)

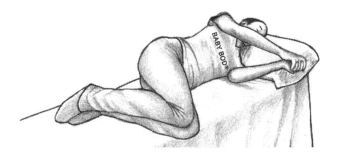

Note: Make sure to use the log roll when moving around and changing positions in bed; try not to twist your back or do a sit-up when you change positions.

How to Safely Sit Up in Bed

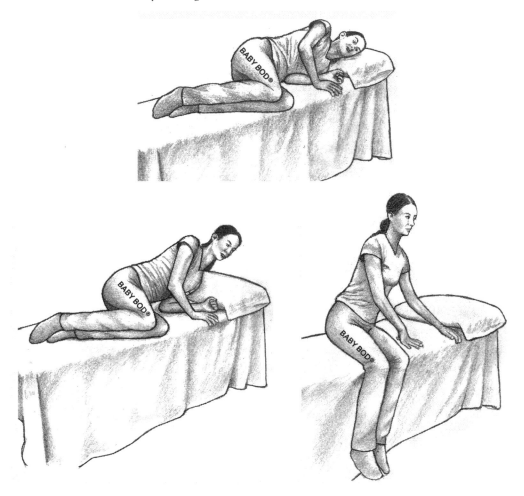

1. After you do the *log roll*, make sure you are at the edge of the bed. *Gently* **EXHALE** and push up with your arms; use the arm that's on top to give you leverage, and use the lower elbow to push down as you lift your body up sideways (as you see in the illustration above).

2. Once you are partially up, drop your legs over the side of the bed so they swing downwards as you continue to push yourself up into a seated position. *Continue exhaling* as you are getting up. Try not to twist your back as you are coming up.

How to Get Up from a Bed (or Chair)

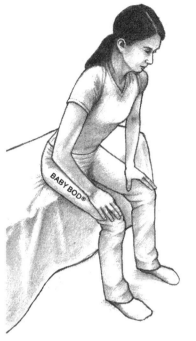

Here is an easy way to take the pressure off your abdominal and pelvic floor muscles when you get up from bed or a chair. This is a good habit to continue to protect your abdominal muscles throughout your entire postpartum recovery.

1. Scoot to the edge of the bed. Make sure you are sitting far enough so your feet are firmly touching the floor.

2. Once you are sitting on the very edge of the bed, lean forward and put the weight of your body on your feet and place your hands on your thighs.

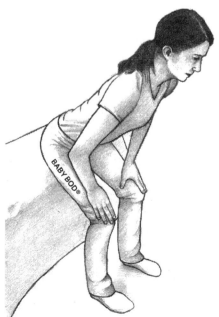

3. To get up, bend forward, and push down on your thighs as you *gently* **EXHALE**, and lift your buttock upwards and off the bed.

4. Use your arm and leg strength to get yourself up. Keep the bent forward position as you continue to get up off the bed. Once you have all the weight on your feet, stand upright.

EXTERNAL SUPPORT FOR THE ABDOMEN AND PELVIS AFTER CHILDBIRTH (VAGINAL DELIVERY)

After birth, women's tummies and pelvic floors need extra support. As I said in previous chapters, the connective tissue and muscles in the abdomen and pelvic floor are stretched out and weak. You can help support them by wearing *medical-grade graduated compression* garments with **LIGHT** compression—I am NOT talking about tight shapewear. Here's what you gain by wearing these while your body is still recovering:

After childbirth, support your tummy by wearing a garment with LIGHT, graduated compression or the Baby Bod® Abdominal Wrap.

+ Light compression increases lymphatic drainage, which will help speed the healing process. Increasing *lymphatic drainage* will also help your body get rid of excess pregnancy fluids faster.

+ Compression will help *decrease your pain.*

+ Elastic helps *muscle memory.* Stretched out muscles will recover faster if you give them a little "assistance." Wearing a garment made out of the *right amount of graduated compression* (*light* medical-grade compression) every day for about three months after childbirth will help your poor stretched out muscles "remember" what it's like to contract and tighten, so they can provide the proper support and hold your internal organs in place.[3, 4, 5]

Just a word of caution: DO NOT make the mistake of thinking you can use the tight shapewear you might already have as a "good enough" or economical alternative. The compression in shapewear garments is too tight and will take over the work of the stomach muscles, which will ultimately weaken your abdominal muscles and prevent you from developing a flat tummy. (Of course, you can still use shapewear garments for a few hours at a time on special occasions, but not all day or as a "postpartum fix.")

So what garments are best? I'll describe them below. I also urge you to go to my website, *www.BabyBodBook.com*, to look for my latest recommendations. When this book went to press, there were several garments on the market for pregnant and postpartum women that I reviewed but did not like because they either did not have *graduated compression* or because the compression was *too tight*. I do have some to recommend now, however. I am always on the lookout for the latest and greatest products for pregnant and postpartum women and update my information frequently. (If you've found a great postpartum support product, please send me information on it via my website. Let's spread the word to other moms or moms-to-be!)

GARMENTS TO CONSIDER
Baby Bod® Abdominal Wrap:

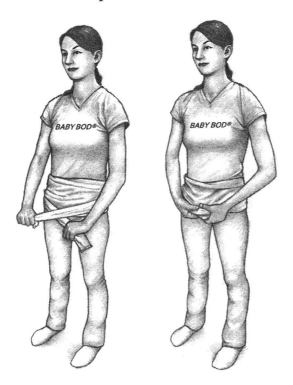

One option to try is the **Baby Bod® Abdominal Wrap**, which you wrap around the pelvis and lower abdomen. For centuries, Mayan women of Central America have used this type of wrap to support the uterus and abdomen for three to four weeks after childbirth. I recommend that you wear it for about a month to six weeks after giving birth; wear it during the day when you are up and about, and not when you sit or sleep. You do have to loosen the wrap each time you sit and readjust it when you get up, so you might not find it as convenient as say, compression shorts. On the other hand, you might find it more comfortable in warmer weather. The wrap can offer just the right amount of support during the early phases of your postpartum recovery. For more information on this, please check my website: *www.BabyBodBook.com*. On the site, you'll also find a video on how to use the **Baby Bod® Abdominal Wrap**.

If you do use the wrap, don't pair it with the compression shorts I describe below. You can alternate them, but don't use them together.

Medical-Grade Compression Shorts:

Another option is a *long-waisted medical-grade compression undergarment* made out of *light, graduated compression material* starting the day after delivery. The ideal garment should look like a pair of shorts with a long waist that goes up to just below your breasts. The compression should be stronger at the bottom of the shorts and lighter at the top. As my research has shown, here is what's ideal: the bottom of the shorts should offer 15 mmHG of compression, which gradually reduces to 12 mmHG of compression by the time you get to the top of the garment.[5] There are not many shorts that provide light, medical-grade, graduated compression, so make sure you do your research before you buy.

Wear them daily if you can, under your clothing, for ten to twelve hours per day for **at least six to eight weeks** after you deliver your child. Do not sleep in them.

Elastic Tee Shirt:

Yet another option is to wear a light elastic tee shirt or camisole that offers *medical-grade graduated compression* similar to that in the shorts. The ideal compression should be a little stronger at the bottom of the tee shirt (around 15 mmHG) and gradually lessen towards the top (around 12 mmHG just under the bust line).

When you consider investing in compression garments, realize that you can wear these long beyond the initial six weeks to eight weeks. Some women continue to use compressive garments on a daily basis for as long as three months, especially if they have diastasis recti.[B] Since the type of garment I recommend is made out of light compression material, you will not run the risk of weakening your abdominal muscles. If you are breastfeeding and you have diastasis recti, consider using the compression garments when you are doing physically demanding activities for the entire time you are breastfeeding—no matter how long that is—AND for the first few months after you STOP breastfeeding. That will give your body some extra support as your hormones get back to normal, which has to happen to allow the connective tissue in your abdomen to stiffen up again. You don't have to wear them all day after the first few months, but do put on your compression garments when you are exercising, lifting or carrying heavy things, or when you have to stand on your feet for long periods of time.

Two Compression Garments to Avoid

Not all compression garments can be used as a postpartum "Mommy Tummy" fix. I already explained why you shouldn't substitute shapewear for garments with light, medical grade compression. Here are two more such garments I urge you to avoid:

Abdominal Binders: "Say NO to tight Abdominal Binders!"

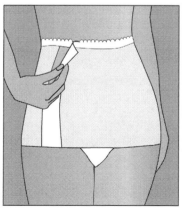

Yoko Design/Shutterstock.com

[B] Diastasis recti is the separation of the abdominal muscles and is common in postpartum women. To read more about diastasis recti, please turn back to Chapter 10.

Say NO to abdominal binders. They squeeze too hard and take over the work of the abdominal muscles, which will ultimately make them weaker. To flatten your postpartum tummy, you need to *strengthen*—not *weaken*—your abdominals! Abdominal binders will NOT permanently flatten your tummy; in the long term, they will do the opposite and make that "Mommy Tummy" worse.

You may hear about these from celebrity moms or well-meaning health and fitness professionals who apparently lack a full understanding of how a woman's core muscles work. There are now a few companies and even a bestselling book that advises women to use tight abdominal binders to develop a flat tummy after childbirth. But I say STEER CLEAR.

Note: *There may be some circumstances where it is medically necessary to use an **elastic binder**.* If you fall into this category, please discuss this information on binders with your healthcare professional. Don't buy or use a binder before you have this discussion.

Elastic Abdominal or "Belly" Bands

For now, say no to elastic abdominal bands. The elastic abdominal bands I found on the market were not made out of graduated compression material and many of them were too tight. So let me caution you: Even though these garments look much more comfortable, they can actually cause more harm than good by potentially causing your abdominal muscles to become weaker over time.

Pelvic/Sacroiliac (SI) Belt:

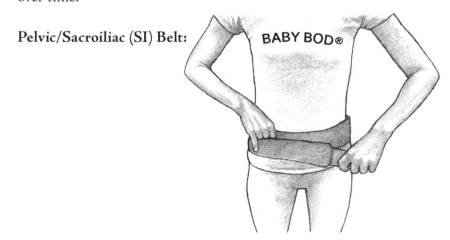

You can begin using a Pelvic/Sacroiliac Belt a day or two after you give birth. This belt sits below the waist and wraps around your pelvic bones and offers additional support to your unstable pelvis and weak core muscles. (After childbirth, the pelvis is often "unstable" and a Pelvic/SI Belt can be useful in preventing pain as well as improving overall function.) You can use it during your everyday activities or to give you extra support when you are trying to progress in your exercise program. Some women find it helpful to use when they sleep to prevent feeling pain when they roll over in bed or get up from bed. (**Note**: It can be used in conjunction with the compression shorts—wear the belt over the shorts—but it will not work over the **Baby Bod® Abdominal Wrap**.)

The **Straight Leg Raise – Core Stability Test** will help you determine if you are a good candidate for a Pelvic/SI Belt. You'll find this test in Chapter Five. If you had a Grade 3 or 4 tear or an episiotomy, however, you must wait until after you have had your six-week postpartum checkup *and* you also must have medical clearance to exercise before performing this test. My best advice for these moms is to try one on and see if you feel like that support is helpful. (For more detailed instructions on Pelvic/SI Belts, please refer to *www.BabyBodBook.com*.)

Pelvic Floor Support Belts:

Pelvic Floor Support Belts are used to give an upward lift and support to the bottom of the pelvis. They can help in healing after childbirth by supporting the pelvic floor and allowing the soft tissue time to heal while in a supported position. These belts were originally designed to reduce the pain caused by varicose veins in the bottom of the pelvis; but they can also be used to control postpartum pain in the perineum. The upward lift should help reduce pain. Some women have told me that these belts also help to decrease the "falling out" feeling[C] they experienced right after childbirth because

---

[C] The "falling out" feeling is often a symptom of pelvic organ prolapse, which was discussed extensively in Chapter 7. If you do have this feeling, please make sure to report it to your doctor or midwife.

the belt helps to "lift the bottom of the pelvis upwards" and offers additional support to the pelvic organs.

You can start using a Pelvic Floor Support Belt one or two days after delivery, as long as it does not cause increased pain where you had a tear or episiotomy. To make the belt more comfortable, try using a sanitary pad between your pelvic floor and the belt.

WHEN IS IT SAFE TO START EXERCISING AGAIN?

Most women are told to REST during the first six weeks after childbirth. And that is exactly what I used to tell my clients up until about five years ago, mostly because I didn't want to go against what the doctor or midwife was recommending. But then I realized that this isn't what's best for new mothers. **It is perfectly safe and beneficial for *most* new moms to start a very gentle exercise program immediately after childbirth.**

When Should YOU Start?

If you've had a vaginal delivery without complications, you can start (or resume) the **Baby Bod® Preliminary Phase Exercises** a day or two after you've had your baby. You'll find these exercises in Chapters Eleven to Fourteen.

Modified Preliminary Phase Exercises – Grade 3 or 4 Tears

If you have a large tear in your perineum or inside your vagina, one that is considered a Grade 3 or 4 tear, you will need to delay starting the "Kegel-like" exercise called the *Pelvic-Core Starter* until after you've had your six-week check-up and gotten medical clearance to resume an exercise program. If you required stitches after delivery, it does not mean you automatically have a Grade 3 or 4 tear (see box below). It is best to ask your midwife or doctor how deep your tear is and how they would grade it. I will explain more in the chapter that covers the *Pelvic-Core Starter*.

Also, if you had a Grade 3 or 4 tear, you must wait until you are six-weeks postpartum and have been given medical clearance before doing the **Straight Leg Raise – Core Stability Test** and the **Diastasis Test**. (See more information on these tests below.)

Perineal and Vaginal Tears

- Many women develop a tear in the perineum (the area between the vagina and anus) and/or vagina during childbirth. It is more common with first-time moms. The amount of tissue that is torn is measured in grades, which can range from a minor cut to a deep laceration that can involve the pelvic floor muscles and/or anal sphincter (the muscles that surround your anus).

- **Grade One** is a superficial tear that can occur in the perineum and or the outermost tissue inside and around the opening to the vagina; a Grade One does not involve the pelvic floor muscles.

- **Grade Two** is a little bit deeper and involves some of the pelvic floor muscle tissue. It needs to be stitched closed and can take a few weeks to heal.

- **Grade Three** can occur in the vagina, perineum and the pelvic floor muscles and can extend to the anal sphincter. It will require stiches to close and will take several weeks to heal. During that time, certain precautions must be taken while the scar tissue forms.

- **Grade Four** is a larger tear that continues through the anal sphincter. It requires stitching and may take longer to heal. During that time, certain precautions must be taken while the scar tissue forms.

What About Walking?

Initially, take two ten-minute walks a day and gradually build up to one thirty-minute walk a few times per week. On the days you cannot walk for thirty minutes, make sure to get in a few ten-minute walks.

For the first six weeks, I also want you to try your best to avoid inclines or uneven surfaces when you're walking outdoors. Then gradually return to walking on all surfaces after your six-week checkup.

When you are trying to return to certain activities, you may find a Pelvic/SI Belt useful in preventing pain in the pelvis and lower back. In fact, many moms find it especially helpful during the first several postpartum months when they use an elliptical machine or do any kind of workout that uses an incline or uneven surfaces. They find that it provides the additional support their body needs until they build up their core strength again.

SIMPLE SELF-ASSESSMENT TESTS

Straight Leg Raise – Core Stability Test

WORKSHEET

If you've had an uncomplicated vaginal delivery, you can do this test soon after giving birth. If you have **large tears (Grade 3 or 4), an episiotomy**, or had a **C-section**, you will need to wait until after your six-week checkup before doing this test. The purpose to this self-test is two-fold. It will help you learn how well your core muscles are stabilizing your torso and whether you would benefit from using a Pelvic/SI Belt.

Turn back to Chapter Five to learn how to do the stability test, and record your results in the worksheet.

Diastasis Recti Test

This is a test to see if the connective tissue that lies in the space between your "six pack" abdominal muscles (the rectus abdominis) is taut enough to hold in your tummy. When the connective tissue is loose, it can cause an unsightly "Mommy Tummy."

You may do this test as early as forty-eight hours after you had an uncomplicated vaginal delivery. If you've had large **vaginal or pelvic floor tear(s) (Grade 3 or 4), an episiotomy or a C-section**, you must wait about six weeks before you do this test. Wait until you have medical clearance to exercise after your six-week checkup.

Please find the diastasis recti test in Chapter Seven. Then record your results on the worksheet.

The Benefits of an Immediate Postpartum Visit with a Physical Therapist

I wrote **Baby Bod**® so that you, at the very least, would have a "virtual physical therapist" and evidence-based advice. But if you want ideal care, you'd do well to make an appointment with a physical therapist for a postpartum visit soon after you give birth.

It's not the norm to visit a physical therapist for a checkup within a week of giving birth, but it should be. This is the best way to ensure that your bones and muscles are aligned and working optimally so that healing can occur as quickly as nature intends. I have long encouraged my pregnant clients to come and see me for a postpartum checkup soon after they deliver their baby, hopefully within a week or so after the delivery. The ones who have taken my suggestion have typically enjoyed a smoother and quicker recovery.

During your postpartum checkup, your therapist might do a few manual therapy treatments, or see if you need additional support anywhere, such as the kind of support a Pelvic/SI Belt can provide. You will also be able to go over the **Baby Bod**® **Preliminary Exercises**, so be sure to bring your book and ask your therapist to check to see if you are doing the exercises correctly. Then it would be best to go back to your physical therapist after you are about six to eight weeks postpartum for a re-evaluation. At that time, you will be able to make a game plan for the most efficient recovery possible. If you are in pain, you may need to see your therapist a few times before the six to eight-week postpartum re-evaluation.

DO SELF-MASSAGE TO SPEED THE HEALING PROCESS

Self-massage is a simple way to help yourself feel better quickly. Any mom can benefit from the **Baby Bod®** self-massages below. Even if it has been months or years since you delivered your child, you can still benefit from doing self-massages. These massages can be used to ease the discomfort caused by common postpartum conditions, such as constipation, diastasis recti, and pain in the abdomen and perineal area. [6, 7] You'll find these easy to do and very beneficial.

The massages I am going to give you are progressive. When you are doing the massage, do not cause pain. There may be some initial discomfort when you first start, but you should not press so hard that you cause pain or a burning sensation along the scar. In time you will be able to progress by using deeper pressure, but you should do that only when you can tolerate it. Don't force it; more is not better.

Abdominal Massages

Massaging the abdomen will help speed up the healing process and improve the ability of the abdominal muscles to start working again.

I am going to teach you three types of abdominal massages: The first one, Abdominal Massage Circles and Skin Rolling, helps to improve blood flow and healing. The second one is geared towards preventing constipation, and the last one helps to recover from diastasis recti.

Moms who have had a vaginal delivery can begin doing Abdominal Massages right after delivery, however, please follow the progression I provide below. You will probably want to wait a few days until you feel less sore. Make sure to start off by using gentle pressure; do NOT cause pain when you massage. Gradually build up the amount of pressure you use as you can tolerate it. During the first few weeks, use the Abdominal Massage Circles, Diastasis Recti Massage and Constipation Massage ONLY. After that time has passed, please add the Skin Rolling Massage. Feel free to do these massages as you watch TV or while listening to music.

Week One
Abdominal Massage Circles

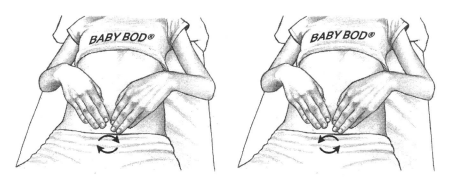

+ Place your two hands together and straighten your fingers. Gently press the pads of your fingers along your panty line, below your belly button.

+ Start on one side of the abdomen and move towards the other side as you do the massage. (See illustration above.)

+ Press down lightly and start with very gentle, circular strokes, first in a clockwise direction, and then in a counterclockwise direction. Do not cause pain. You should feel a gentle pull in your skin as your move your fingers in circular motions.

+ Do this for about a minute.

+ Then move your fingers to the middle of your abdomen, on your panty line, right below your belly button and repeat as above.

+ Then move your fingers again to the other side of your abdomen and continue massaging for about a minute.

+ Then move your fingers to about 2 inches (5cm) above your belly button and repeat the same massage in three different areas, one to the side of the belly button, one in the middle, and one to the other side of the belly button.

+ Do this for a total of 6 minutes per day for one week and then progress to the Stage Two massage instructions.

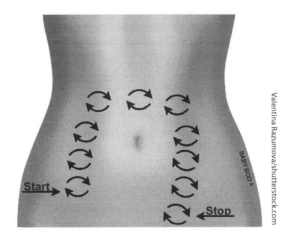

Constipation Massage Path

Constipation Massage [8]

The self-massage for constipation is simple and easy to perform. If you had a vaginal delivery, you can do it as early as a day or so after you delivered your child. It consists of circular motions applied over a path of approximately ten spots in your lower abdomen, to help move the bowel content.

+ Lie down in a comfortable spot like your bed. Place a pillow beneath your knees.

+ Place 2-3 fingers in the lower right side of your abdomen (refer to the illustration above), over the first massage spot, and gently apply a constant and moderate pressure. If you experience pain, lighten up the pressure. Then maintain this pressure as you move your fingers in **clockwise, circular**

motions for approximately 10 seconds. (**Note:** Do not use counterclockwise strokes.)

+ Move to the next massage spot and repeat as above.

+ Gradually continue the clockwise massage circles up towards your rib cage, then across to the left side of your abdomen, and down to the inner-left side of your pelvis. Each massage path should last a total of 1 minute.

+ Repeat the entire massage path from your right side to your left side a few times, once a day.

Weeks Two to Twelve

Abdominal Massage Circles

Continue the massage in all six areas on your tummy as you did in week one, but this time press a little bit harder, but not so hard that it causes pain. Alternate clockwise and counterclockwise massage strokes for a total of 6 minutes. Do this for one week and then continue to increase the amount of pressure over the next 12 weeks, but only up to the point before you experience pain. If you feel pain, ease back.

Self-Massage for Diastasis Recti

Did you know that self-massage can help you heal diastasis recti? (Please refer to Chapter Seven to learn more about diastasis recti.) In my clinic, the women who learn and do this massage often recover faster and are able to "activate" their core muscles more easily. You can start doing this massage a few days after you deliver your baby if you had a vaginal delivery.

Make sure not to press so hard that it causes pain. If you feel pain in specific spots, that is not so unusual. Just lighten up the pressure in the painful spots as you do the massage.

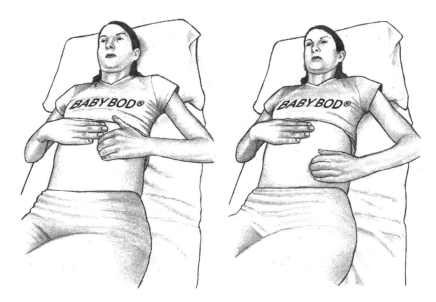

Diastasis Recti Masssage

+ Place a flat hand on your tummy at the bottom of your ribcage. Press down gently to secure the skin as you do the massage with your other hand. (Refer to the illustrations above.)

+ Keep the fingers on your other hand together. Place your fingers about 3 inches (7-8cm) away from the midline of the abdomen (please refer to the picture). This hand will be massaging one side of the rectus abdominis muscle.

+ Gently press into the skin and maintain this pressure as you move your fingers downwards toward your panty line. It should feel as if you are "pulling" your skin downwards. You may even feel a slight burning sensation as you pull the skin, which is the effect you are going for. Although this is normal, do not press so hard that you cause pain beyond that slight burning sensation.

+ Do this about 10 times on each side of your tummy, every day, until your diastasis goes away.

Weeks Four to Twelve
  Abdominal Massage Circle - Continue as directed earlier.
  Self-Massage for Diastasis Recti - Continue as directed earlier.

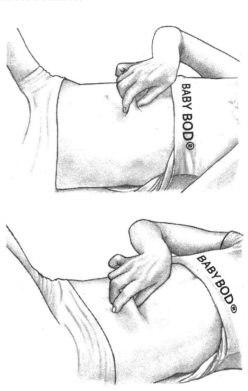

Abdominal Skin Rolling Massage

When you are about four weeks postpartum, continue doing the Abdominal Massage Circles as described above and add the Skin Rolling Massage.[D] (Do not start this massage before you are four weeks postpartum.)

- To roll your skin, gently grab a roll of skin in the upper part of your abdomen between your fingers and thumb.

- Then move the skin roll down towards your panty line. To do this, use your thumb to push the skin roll towards your pubic bone. Your fingers should "walk" towards your panty line as you push the roll with your thumb. Do not cause pain. (See the illustrations.)

- Do this along the middle of your tummy, then down the right side and then the left side.

- Try to do this for 1 to 2 minutes.

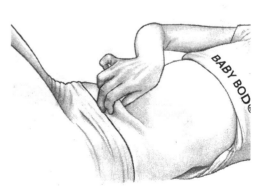

Abdominal Skin Rolling Massage

[D] Skin rolling can be very uncomfortable. If you find it painful, lighten up on your pressure by pulling less skin into the roll and don't press as hard with your fingers.

Pelvic Floor Massages

After childbirth, many women are left with tears (lacerations) in the pelvic floor and or inside the vagina. These areas often require stitches and form into scars as they heal. You can help Mother Nature along by performing the two perineal (pelvic floor) massages below (after your six-week checkup). [7]

The first massage is for scar tissue that was caused by tears or an episiotomy, and the second one can help to relieve pelvic pain caused by "trigger points" in muscles. Please wait until after you have had your six-week checkup and have been told that you have fully healed by your midwife or doctor before doing these massages.

Perineal Scar Tissue Rolling

This is helpful to use on scars caused by a tear or an episiotomy in the perineum and pelvic floor muscles. Wait until you have been given medical clearance after your six-week checkup before doing a Perineal Massage. (You have to make sure that the scar has healed before you start to massage it. I also advise you to use a massage lubricant when you do this massage.)

Here is how to do it:

+ Gently hold the scar tissue between your fingertips, as if you are gently pinching a roll of skin.

+ Gently "roll" the scar between your fingers tips for 1 to 2 minutes. Make sure to change the areas you are holding and move up and down the length of the scar.

+ Do this for a minute or two on each scar.

+ Continue doing this daily until the scar feels softer and more flexible and is pain free.

Pelvic Floor Trigger Point Massage

This is a great way to relieve pain in the perineum, vagina and pelvic floor muscles. It might help make sex less painful too. Please wait until you are six weeks postpartum before doing the Trigger Point Massage. You can use an "S-shaped massage wand" or your finger to do a Trigger Point Massage. (You can find a massage wand on our website or by Googling "pelvic floor massage wand.")

- Use gentle finger pressure to find a spot that is painful in you perineum, the area between your vagina and anus or on the sides of your pelvic floor. You may also find painful spots inside your vagina.

- Once you locate a painful spot (trigger point), gently press into the painful trigger point with your finger or the massage wand and hold it there for about 2 minutes.

  - Make sure not to press too hard; it should feel as if you are causing the pain to increase a little, not a lot. As you continue to press, the pain should start to decrease. If the pain increases, either lighten up the amount you are pressing or skip that area and try it again in a day or two.

- Then continue looking for more painful spots (trigger points). Press into the new trigger point for about 2 minutes and release (as above).

- Try to alternate and press the trigger points at different angles when you repeat it the next day.

- Try to do this on a daily basis until the pain and tenderness goes away.

  - **Note:** Instead of using your finger, you can try this with an **"S-shaped" massage wand** that is designed for this purpose.

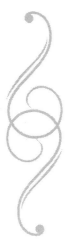

Self-Care Summary for Moms Who Had a Vaginal Delivery

Try to:

1. Avoid placing extra strain on your abdominal and pelvic floor muscles by avoiding any movements that resemble a sit-up or crunch. (Read more about the negative effects of sit-ups in Chapter Ten.)

2. Reduce pain by applying **iced gloves**, using a **sitz bath** and a **peri bottle**.

3. Get out of bed as soon as you have medical clearance and **walk** around a bit.

4. Prevent **constipation** by adding enough fiber to your diet and using **good toilet posture** (as discussed in Chapter Seven.)

5. Use **external support** such as the **Baby Bod® Abdominal Wrap**, or a garment made out of medical grade graduated compression material to reduce pain and speed healing. Other helpful garments are the Pelvic/SI Belt and the Pelvic Floor Support Belt.

6. Start the **Preliminary Phase** of the **Baby Bod® Program** a day or so after delivery.

7. Use a **pillow to support the baby** when you nurse or bottle-feed your child.

8. Do the **abdominal self-massages** (as described above) a few days after delivery.

9. Start doing the **perineal massages** after your six-week checkup.

10. Avoid **holding your breath** whenever you exert yourself.

I hope you're basking in the glow of your accomplishment and enjoying all those bonding moments with your new baby instead of wondering why your empty belly still looks like a slightly deflated basketball. PATIENCE…You *will* get that flat tummy back. In the meantime, stay off the scale. (See "Why the Scale Hasn't Budged Yet" in Chapter Two.) And do remember to make time for your twice-daily walks, which will make the numbers on the scale look way better once it's time to look at it again.

The walks are part of the overall exercise program, which you will learn next. Please skip the next chapter, which is for women who have had a C-section, and go directly to Chapter Ten.

And do remember to make time for your twice-daily walks.

[1] Renfrew MJ, Lang S. Do cabbage leaves prevent breast engorgement? A randomized, controlled study. *Birth*. 1993;20:2. doi: 10.1111/j.1523-536X.1993.tb00418.x.

[2] Roberts KL, Reiter M, Schuster D. A comparison of chilled and room temperature cabbage leaves in treating breast engorgement. *Journal of Human Lactation*. 1995. 11(3): 191-4. doi: 10.1177/089033449501100319

[3] Sawan S, Mugnai R, de Barros Lopes A, et al. Lower-Limb Lymphedema and Vulval Cancer: Feasibility of Prophylactic Compression Garments and Validation of Leg Volume Measurement. *Int J Gynecol Cancer*. December 2009; 19(9):1649-1654; doi: 10.1111/IGC.0b013e3181a8446a.

[4] Cheifetz O, Lucy SD, Overend TJ, Crowe J. The Effect of Abdominal Support on Functional Outcomes in Patients Following Major Abdominal Surgery: A Randomized Controlled Trial. *Physiotherapy Can*. 2010 Summer; 62(3):242–253. doi:10.3138/physio.62.3.242.

[5] Annoni F, Pasche P, Torre R, De Stefano A, Annoni GA, Lucci C. Class 2 Compression Stockings According to ENC Standard with Innovative Features. *Minerva Cardioangiologica*. 2006; 54(3).

[6] Lewit K, Olsanske S. Clinical Importance of active scars: abnormal scars as and the cause of myofacial pain. *J Manipulative Physiol Ther*. 2004, 27(6): 399-402. http://www.eugenept.com/pdfs/clinicaimprtance.pdf

[7] Arung W, Meurisse M, Detry O. Pathophysiology and prevention of postoperative peritoneal adhesions. *World J Gastroenterol*. 2011; 17(41): 4545-4553. doi: 10.3748/wjg.v17.i41.4545.

[8] McClurg D, Lowe-Strong A. Does abdominal massage relieve constipation? *Nursing Times*. 2011.107(12):20-22. http://www.nursingtimes.net/Journals/2013/01/18/m/y/j/290311Does-abdominal-massage-relieve-constipation.pdf

Self-Care After a C-Section

If you're among the one-third of moms in the U.S.—or the many moms elsewhere—who have given birth by Cesarean section, know that you, too, can safely do **Baby Bod®**. If you had your C-section recently, however, you may need to wait a little longer to start some aspects of it. (I'll address that in more detail below and help you tailor the program for you.)

Having a C-section is no picnic, especially in the beginning. After enduring so many uncomfortable changes during pregnancy—and then major surgery—you're looking forward to getting your body back to normal. This doesn't happen instantly, something you know full well if this isn't your first C-section. You do have to be patient as Nature takes its course, but there are *smart* ways to help Nature along. Knowing *WHAT to do WHEN* and *WHAT NOT to do* can make a big difference.

In this chapter, I'll talk about how you can make yourself more comfortable in the immediate aftermath of surgery and how to get a great start on healing the scar left by your incision. These steps will put your recovery into high gear. If, by chance, you're starting **Baby Bod®** months after you've given birth, however, you can skip most of it, but do make sure to do the self-tests and massages, which are described further down in this chapter. It's never too late to benefit from those.

Let's start with some general tips.

Tip # 1: Cut Yourself a Break

On the off chance you don't know this, a C-section is considered major surgery. Recovering from any kind of major surgery takes time. So think about how much you're asking of your body when you expect it to recover quickly even though you're caring for your

Knowing what to do when and what not to do can make a big difference.

baby around the clock. In addition, you're going through the same postpartum changes every mother has to go through.

Remember that your abdominal and pelvic floor muscles need time to heal. As I said in Chapter Five, it takes—on average—about six weeks to complete just the *first stage* of soft tissue (connective tissue) healing after delivery. It will take at least *another six to eight weeks* for your ligaments and connective tissue to return to "normal" if you are not breastfeeding. (That is a total of THREE months after childbirth.) If you are breastfeeding, however, it can take up to *three months after you stop nursing* for your connective tissue to regain the ability to support your body like it did before you got pregnant.

If you don't go easy on yourself and you strain your muscles during this period, recovery will take that much longer. This is why you need to be patient with yourself and your recovery process. Don't even think about jumping back into your regular routine right away! Embrace a gradual recovery.

At minimum, take off six weeks from work; make it at least three months if you possibly can. (More time off from work is even better.)

When you first get home from the hospital, pay close attention to how you feel. Don't hesitate to call your doctor if you are in pain, have excessive bleeding, find it difficult to breathe, or start to develop a fever or dizziness. And yes, *follow your doctor's orders*[A] (with the one exception I will give you in Tip #3 below).

Tip # 2: Get Help with Taxing Household Tasks

As I said earlier, arrange for help with household tasks that are physically taxing, like grocery shopping and housework. Don't be afraid to ask. Have someone else do the heavy lifting when setting up—or re-arranging—the nursery. And imprint this one rule in your brain: Do not lift or push anything heavier than your newborn baby for the first six weeks after you had your baby.

This includes carrying grocery bags, strollers, laundry baskets and the like. Also, try to avoid pushing a vacuum cleaner or opening

Do not lift or push anything heavier than your newborn baby for the first 6 weeks after you had your baby.

[A] Your doctor will give you instructions on how to care for your incision and on the activities you can and can't do, before you leave the hospital.

heavy doors until you reach the six-week postpartum benchmark. (In Chapter Seventeen, I'll talk more about how to move around safely with as little strain as possible.)

Tip # 3: Carve Out Time to Learn the Baby Bod® Preliminary Phase Exercises

Most doctors will caution you not to exercise for six weeks to allow your body to heal from surgery. You might be surprised to learn that you can safely return to some gentle exercises, as early as the day after you had your C-section. I will lay them out for you in this program. However, I do want you to check with your doctor—just to be on the safe side—before starting the **Baby Bod® Preliminary Phase Exercises.** Show your doctor the gentle exercises in the program during one of your prenatal visits, or when you are recovering in the hospital, and ask if these are okay for you in your current condition. You can also consult your doctor about the pain-relieving tips (are there any that aren't advisable for you?) and ask the best time to start the self-massages. Just be sure to explain to your doctor that the exercises you plan to do have been specifically designed by a physical therapist for women who have had C-sections. (If you just ask your doctor, "Can I exercise?" you're likely to get an outright no.)

Let me explain why I don't advocate *complete* rest after a C-section—except for those of you with pregnancy-related disorders or postoperative complications where complete rest is appropriate. Your body needs to move to keep the blood circulating, which is an important part of the healing process. If you are too sedentary, it interrupts the normal flow of blood to the tissues, which can delay healing and make you feel stiff and tired. **The Baby Bod® Preliminary Phase Exercises** will help get your circulation going and bring many other benefits besides.

If you start them soon after you deliver your baby, you get a jump-start because you start six weeks earlier than most other moms. Those first six weeks will help your muscles become "awake and ready" for the more progressive strengthening exercises that follow, so you'll also get better results than moms who haven't done the necessary work to fully recover their core muscles. Then, after you have your six-week checkup and get the "all clear" signal from your doctor, you may do some of the tests that are in Chapter Five (the Straight Leg Raise Test and Diastasis Recti Test) and progress to the advanced exercises and abdominal massages with no restrictions.

DAY-BY-DAY HEALING GUIDE

If you've had a Cesarean section, the chart below will tell you when you can safely begin individual components of the **Baby Bod® Program.** Meanwhile, here are some things that can keep you comfortable immediately after you give birth[B]:

+ At least 2 dozen **non-latex gloves.** (You'll pack these with ice and use them for pain relief.)
+ Microwavable **moist heating pads.** These will be handy to relieve neck and lower back pain. Use the pads for 15 minutes at a time.
+ Special items that can help support your body, such as the **Baby Bod® Abdominal Wrap, medical-grade compression shorts** with a **long waist,** a **Pelvic/SI Belt*** and possibly a **Pelvic Floor Support Belt*.** I'll talk about these in a bit.
+ A **small (12" by 12") pillow**— if you had a Cesarean birth, you'll find it helpful to hold this pillow against your tummy when you cough, roll over in bed, or get out of bed.
+ **Two tennis balls inside a tube sock** to be used to roll over sore muscles.
+ **A donut-shaped pillow** to sit on.
+ **Sitz bath**
+ **Peri bottle**

*Unlike mothers who had a vaginal delivery, you will need to wait a couple of weeks before using a **Pelvic/SI Belt** or a **Pelvic Floor Support Belt.**

[B] If the list looks familiar, it's because I mentioned these in an earlier chapter for pregnant women.

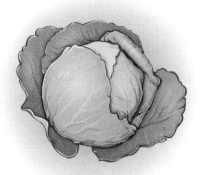

Codrut Crososchi/Shutterstock.com

Do Cabbage Leaves Relieve Pain? Or Is That a Myth?

Many new mothers report that making a compress of fresh cabbage leaves and placing it on their breasts helps relieve the pain of engorgement. I never tried this myself, but you might want to give it a go.

A study done by the Cochrane Pregnancy and Childbirth Group showed that cabbage leaves can help to relieve the discomfort and pain many women experience during the engorgement phase, although researchers are not absolutely sure why. [1] Mothers who do this boil the cabbage, then let it cool down to room temperature or chill it. Then they crush it so that the veins on the leaves are broken. They place a few crushed leaves on the breast for about twenty minutes and apply the compress three to four times a day during the engorgement phase. [2]

This is probably safe to try unless you are allergic to sulfa drugs because the cabbage leaves contain sulfa. So if you have a sulfa drug allergy, steer clear. (If you are not sure whether you can tolerate sulfa, try doing a "skin patch test" by putting a piece of boiled cabbage on your forearm for twenty-four hours first.)

SELF-CARE CHART

Here's a chart you can start using right after you deliver your child and continue to use for a couple of months.

Note: The garments listed in the chart below are *suggestions* to help support your body during the healing phase. You may find them helpful for months and even years after childbirth. Most moms pick and choose which supportive garments work best for them.

HEALING TIMELINE * * *	C-section
What to Do...	**When to Start...**
Ice-packed gloves on incision and pelvic floor if sore	Start to use it on the pelvic floor area right after birth if you have pain. Wait a few days after delivery to use ice on your incision; get medical clearance first.
Ankle exercises in bed	Right after delivery
Sitz bath	24 hours after delivery (if necessary to relieve pain): get medical clearance first.
Walk	Within 24 hours. (Get medical clearance first. You may need to wait until after your bladder catheter is removed. Do not try to get up on your own; your nurse, physical therapist or doula should be there to assist you the first time you get out of bed.)
Modified Preliminary Phase Exercises (you'll find these in Chapters 11-14). See chart on page 172 for the modified version.	24-48 hours after delivery
Compressive stockings	Right after delivery. (You will be provided with a pair in the hospital.)
Baby Bod® Abdominal Wrap – wear 10 to 12 hours a day, especially to be worn when you are up and about. Remove or loosen when you are sitting down.	24 hours after delivery
Long-waisted medical-grade compression shorts. Wear 10 – 12 hours per day. (See more information below.)	48 hours after delivery. (You may need to wait a few more days, until you feel comfortable wearing them.)

HEALING TIMELINE * * * (continued)	C-section
Pelvic/SI Belt for support, if it helps, when you're up and about. (In Chapter 5 you'll find a quick self-test, the Straight Leg Raise Test, that will help you determine if you're a candidate for the SI Belt. Wait until after your six-week postpartum checkup to do this test.)	After your stitches are removed and the belt does not irritate the skin (usually 2 or 3 weeks).
Pelvic Floor Support Belt. When necessary, wear when you are up and about for 10 to 12 hours.	After your stitches are removed and the belt does not irritate the skin (usually 2 or 3 weeks).
Straight Leg Raise – Core Stability Test (you'll find this on in Chapter 5)	6 to 8 weeks after delivery. Wait until you have medical clearance to exercise.
Diastasis Recti Test (found in Chapter 7)	6 to 8 weeks. Wait until you have medical clearance to exercise.
Abdominal Massages: 1. Abdominal and Scar Tissue Circles (Progress to Skin Rolling) 2. Diastasis Recti Massage 3. Constipation Massage	Start 6 weeks after delivery, except Skin Rolling. Start Skin Rolling one month after you started the other abdominal massages.

Pelvic Floor Massages (found below):
  1. Perineal Scar tissue Massage
  2. Pelvic Floor Trigger Point Massage
	Start 6 weeks after delivery.

* * * You can find all of these items in the **Baby Bod® Store** at *www.BabyBodBook.com*. You'll find the site useful as a reference, even if get your garments elsewhere.

SELF-CARE IMMEDIATELY AFTER BIRTH – PAIN RELIEF TIPS
Ice Is Nice:

To relieve pain, you can make an ice pack by filling a non-latex glove with ice and apply it to the pelvic floor immediately after birth if you have pain in your bottom, but you must have medical clearance before applying it to your incision. (You may need to wait a few days.) Make sure to clean your hands first and wrap the glove with a thin cloth before applying it to your incision or pelvic floor. (Do not apply the ice-filled glove directly on your skin without a thin cloth to protect your skin.) Keep it there for ten to fifteen minutes at a time. Replace the ice glove with a new clean glove and cloth each time. (Using a new glove and cloth will guard against infection.) Try to use the ice packs several times a day when you're feeding or nursing your baby or resting. Continue this practice until the pain goes away.

Other Helpful Tips to Relive Pain:

Here are a few things you can do to *relieve or prevent* aches and pains in your pelvis, back, upper back or neck. ***Try:***

- Using a **sitz bath** 24 hours after delivery to relieve pain in your bottom. (Even though you had a Cesarean section, you might have a sore bottom.) It is a plastic bowl that sits on top of your toilet seat; you will usually be given one during your stay in the hospital. Fill it with lukewarm water and sit in it for about 10 to 15 minutes at a time. The water should feel warm, but not so hot that it burns. You may need to refill the water as you sit on it to keep the temperature warm.

- Sitting on a **donut-shaped pillow.** These come in handy to relieve aches and pains in your perineum and pain from hemorrhoids.

- Using a **peri bottle,** which is made out of flexible plastic, can ease discomfort or stinging when you urinate. Fill the bottle with warm water and squirt it on your bottom as you pee. Then gently pat yourself dry with toilet paper or tissues. Continue to use a peri bottle until the pain or stinging goes away, which could take a few weeks. It is also nice to use to clean the bloody vaginal discharge (lochia) you will be experiencing during the early postpartum days.

- Using a **microwavable heating pad** to relieve muscle tension in your back or neck one or two times a day for about 15 minutes at a time. You can use the pad when you are feeding your baby; that way you will be doing two good things at once.

+ Slipping two **tennis balls** into an old sock and then tying a knot in the sock. Use it as a massage tool to roll over sore muscles. (Don't sit on them.)

+ Learning **good toilet posture** to decrease strain on the pelvic floor. (I covered this in Chapter Seven.)

+ **Preventing constipation**: A lot of new mothers complain of constipation right after childbirth, especially after a C-section. It can take a few days for your bowels to "wake up" after surgery, and pain medication can cause constipation. You may be given a stool softener to take to make it easier to pass a bowel movement and some doctors may prescribe a gentle laxative. Believe it or not, walking will help prevent constipation. The self-massage for constipation I describe below can also help "push things along," but don't start doing it until six weeks after surgery.

+ Using a **small pillow** (about 12 by 12 inches or 30 by 30cm) to reduce pain from the C-section incision. Press it against your tummy when you roll in bed, get up from a chair and when you cough or sneeze. Try pressing a small pillow against your stomach as you try to pass a bowel movement.

+ Wearing **compressive garments** and **Pelvic Support Belts** (after a few weeks), because they may also reduce pain. We will discuss them later in this chapter.

+ Using **good body mechanics** when you move around. Don't be surprised if you experience pain during everyday activities, like rolling in bed or getting out of bed or a chair, for a while after surgery. (Later in this chapter, I'll explain how to do all of this with the least amount of effort or strain on your body.) In Chapters Sixteen and Seventeen, I will give you even more advice on how to protect your body after childbirth.

Walking will help to improve your circulation and prevent constipation.

That said, if you are in pain, DON'T KEEP SILENT. Make sure you discuss this with your doctor, doula or nurse.

Motion Is Lotion:

Right after surgery, you will be told to rest as much as possible, but that doesn't mean you should stay in bed the whole time. The thought of getting out of bed might frighten you; you may feel that you will never be able to walk again. So you may be shocked when your doctor tells you it is time to **get out of bed and walk around the room at first, then down the hospital hallways.** The sooner you start moving, the quicker you will be able to heal and prevent blood clots from forming in your legs. Walking will help to improve your circulation and prevent constipation. You will usually have to wait until a day after surgery, until the bladder catheter is removed, before you can get out of bed. Wait until you have medical clearance and *make sure* there is a medical professional there to assist you the first time you get out of bed.

Until you can start walking around, or in-between walks, it is important to do some **ankle exercises** several times per hour if you are awake. Try to point and flex your foot ten times, then move your feet in circles, ten times clockwise and ten times counterclockwise.

When you return home, remind yourself to move during the day. We physical therapists have a saying: "Motion is lotion." You need to keep your body moving to keep the blood circulating, which keeps your bones and muscles healthy. Movement also increases the healthy fluids in your joints, which will prevent stiffness. When you are sedentary, it interrupts the normal flow of blood to the tissues. That leads to stiffness and feelings of fatigue.

Even small movements can help. When you sit to nurse or feed your baby, or sit at your computer, try to change positions a few times. And when you can't move that much, you can still combat stiffness with small movements like moving your head around to stretch out your neck muscles, rolling your shoulders, or arching and rounding out your back to stretch out your back muscles. In short, move! This will keep you flexible—and energetic.

Moving Around and Sitting Up In Bed:

Here's a sequence you can use to protect your tummy when you are getting up from bed. It takes a few steps to learn this. The first thing you need to realize is that you want to *roll over in bed*—as I will explain—*instead of lifting your body up as if you are doing a sit-up*. (Another name for this is "jackknife behavior.") If you are lying on your back, for instance, do NOT lift your head and chest off the bed first. Instead, use a log roll to roll yourself to the side of the bed, and then push yourself up sideways. And remember to EXHALE as you move around to prevent building up the kind of internal pressure that will make your belly bulge. (I covered this in detail in the earlier chapter on the core muscles.)

How to Roll Over in Bed (Log Roll with Pillow)

Use a pillow with the technique below to help prevent pain.

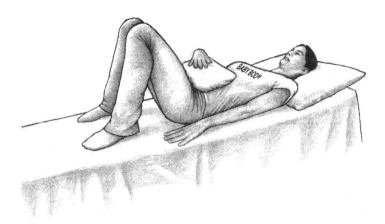

1. Lie on your back with your knees bent. Press the pillow on your tummy, over your incision. Use the hand on the opposite side you are turning towards to hold the pillow. For the purposes of these instructions, let's imagine that's the left side of the bed. If you're rolling to the left, hold the pillow over your incision with your right hand. (*Continues next page.*)

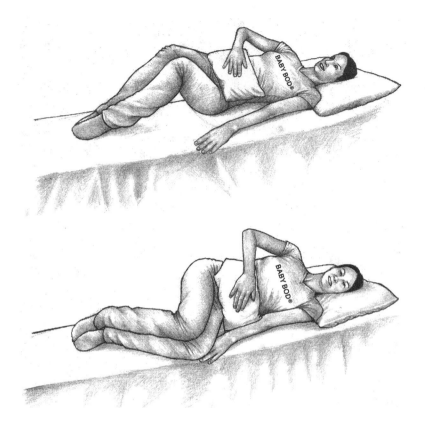

2. Continue pressing, and then gently **EXHALE** (as if you are cleaning sunglasses) as you roll over to your side. Keeping your body straight, try to move your shoulders and pelvis at the same time. (Roll over like a log.)

Note: Make sure to use the log roll when moving around and changing positions in bed; try not to twist your back or do a sit-up when you change positions.

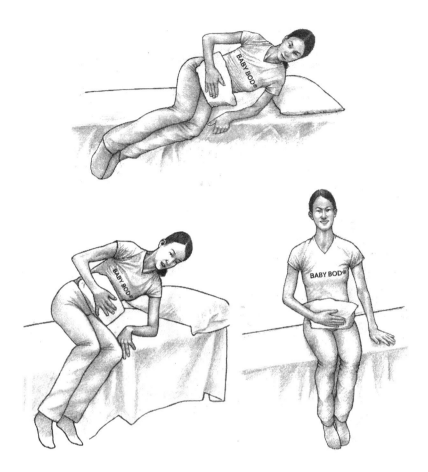

How to Safely Sit Up in Bed

1. After you do the *log roll,* make sure you are at the edge
    of the bed. Continue pressing the pillow with your right
    hand. Then gently EXHALE as you push yourself up
    with your left arm.

2. Once you are partially up, drop your legs over the side of
    the bed so they swing downwards as you continue to push
    yourself up into a seated position. (Don't hold your breath;
    make sure to EXHALE.)

How to Get Up from a Bed (or Chair)

Here is an easy way to take the pressure off your abdominal and pelvic floor muscles when you get up from bed or a chair. This is a good habit to continue to protect your abdominal muscles throughout your entire postpartum recovery.

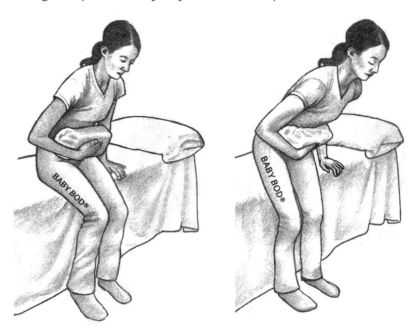

1. To get up from the bed or a chair, first scoot to the edge of the bed. Make sure you are sitting far enough so your feet are firmly touching the floor. Continue pressing the pillow to support your stomach. Once you are sitting on the very edge of the bed, lean forward and put the weight of your body on your feet. Place the hand not holding the pillow on the edge of the bed.

2. To get up, continue pressing the pillow to support your stomach and gently EXHALE. Use your other hand to push yourself up from bed. Keep the bent forward position as you continue to get up off the bed. Once you have all the weight on your feet, stand upright.

EXTERNAL SUPPORT FOR THE ABDOMEN AND THE PELVIS AFTER CHILDBIRTH (C-SECTION)

You will be given a pair of **compressive stockings** that look like knee socks right after surgery. It is important to wear them, as instructed, to help control swelling and prevent blood clots from forming in your legs.

You may also be given an **elastic abdominal binder** to wear after surgery. *I am not a fan of using these for the long term*, for reasons I will explain below. Many women find that using an elastic abdominal binder can help to reduce abdominal pain during the initial week or so after surgery. If you use a binder for longer periods, however, it may work against your recovery.

These aren't the only compression garments that might be helpful in the weeks and months following your C-section. After birth, women's tummies and pelvic floors need extra support. As I said in previous chapters, the connective tissue and muscles in the abdomen and pelvic floor are stretched out and weak. You can help support them by wearing *medical grade compression* **garments with LIGHT compression**[3, 4, 5]—I am NOT talking about tight, tight shapewear. Here's what you gain by wearing these garments while your body is still recovering:

After childbirth, support your tummy by wearing a garment with LIGHT, graduated compression or the Baby Bod® Abdominal Wrap.

+ Light compression increases *lymphatic drainage*, which will help speed the healing process. Increasing lymphatic drainage will also help your body get rid of excess pregnancy fluids faster.

+ Compression will help *decrease your pain*.

+ Elastic helps *muscle memory*. Stretched out muscles will recover faster if you give them a little "assistance." Wearing a garment made out of the *right amount of compression (light* medical grade compression) every day for about three months after childbirth will help your poor stretched out muscles "remember" what it's like to contract and tighten, so they can provide the proper support and hold your internal organs in place.

Just a word of caution: DO NOT make the mistake of thinking you can use the tight shapewear you might already have as a "good enough" or less costly alternative. The compression in shapewear garments is too tight and will take over the work of the stomach muscles, which will ultimately weaken your abdominal muscles and prevent you from developing a flat tummy. (Of course, you can still use shapewear garments for a few hours at a time on special occasions, but not all day or as a "postpartum fix.")

So what garments are best? I'll describe them briefly below. I also urge you to go to my website, *www.BabyBodBook.com*, to look for my latest recommendations. When this book went to press, there were several garments on the market for pregnant and postpartum women that I reviewed but did not like because they either did not have graduated compression or because the compression was too tight. I do have some to recommend now, however. I am always on the lookout for the latest and greatest products for pregnant and postpartum women and update my information frequently. (If you've found a great postpartum support product, please send me information on it via my website. Let's spread the word to other moms or moms-to-be!)

GARMENTS TO CONSIDER
Baby Bod®
Abdominal Wrap:

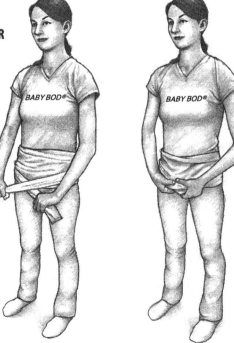

One option to try is the **Baby Bod® Abdominal Wrap**, which you wrap around the pelvis and lower abdomen. For centuries, Mayan women of Central America have used this type of wrap to support the uterus and abdomen for three to four weeks after childbirth. I recommend that you wear it for about a month to six weeks after giving birth; wear it during the day when you are up and about, and not when you sit or sleep. You do have to loosen the wrap each time you sit and readjust it when you get up, so you might not find it as convenient as the shorts I describe below. On the other hand, you might find it more comfortable in warmer weather. The wrap may offer just the right amount of support during the early phases of your postpartum recovery. If you do use the wrap, don't pair it with the compression shorts I describe below. You can alternate them, but don't use them together.

If you use the elastic binder they give you at the hospital, consider alternating it with the **Baby Bod® Abdominal Wrap** when you need to take a break from using the elastic binder. For more information on this, please visit my website: *www.BabyBodBook.com*. On the site, you'll also find a video on how to use the **Baby Bod® Abdominal Wrap**.

If you do use the wrap, don't pair it with the compression shorts I describe below. You can alternate them, but don't use them together.

Medical Grade Compression Shorts:
Another option is *long-waisted medical-grade compression undergarment* made out of *light graduated compression material* starting the day after delivery. The ideal garment should look like a pair of shorts with a long waist that goes up to just below your breasts. The compression should be stronger at the bottom of the shorts and lighter at the top. As my research has shown, here is what's ideal: the bottom of the shorts should offer 15 mmHG of compression, which gradually reduces to 12 mmHG of compression by the time you get to the top of the garment. There are not many shorts that provide light, medical grade, graduated compression, so make sure you do your research before you buy.

You may need to wait a few more days until you feel comfortable wearing them. Try placing a sanitary napkin with the sticky side out over your incision to prevent rubbing against it when you take the shorts on and off. Once the incision is healed, you can stop using the napkin to protect the incision.[C]

Wear them daily if you can, under your clothing, for ten to twelve hours per day for at least six to eight weeks after you deliver your child. Do not sleep in them.

Elastic Tee Shirt:

Yet another option is to wear a light elastic tee shirt or camisole that offers medical-grade graduated compression similar to that in the shorts. The ideal compression should be a little stronger at the bottom of the tee shirt (around 15 mmHG) and gradually lessen towards the top (around12 mmHG just under the bust line).

When you consider investing in compression garments, realize that you can wear these long beyond the initial six weeks to eight weeks. Some women continue to use compressive garments on a daily basis for as long as three months, especially if they have diastasis recti.[D] Since the type of garment I recommend is made out of lightweight compression material, you will not run the risk of weakening your abdominal muscles. If you are breastfeeding and you have diastasis recti, consider using the compression garments when you are doing physically demanding activities for the entire time you are breastfeeding—no matter how long that is—AND for the first few months after you stop breastfeeding. That will give your body some extra support as your hormones get back to normal, which has to happen to allow the connective tissue in your abdomen to stiffen again. You don't have to wear them all day long after the first few months, but do put on your compression garments when you are exercising, lifting, or carrying heavy things, or when you have to stand on your feet for long periods of time.

[C] This great idea was shared by Fiona Rodgers, a physiotherapist from Queensland, Australia. (www.pelvicfloorexercise.com.au)

[D] Diastasis recti is the separation of the abdominal muscles and is common in postpartum women. To read more about diastasis recti, please turn back to Chapter 10.

Two Compression Garments to Avoid

Not all compression garments are good. I already explained why you shouldn't substitute shapewear for garments with light, medical-grade compression. Here are two more such garments I urge you to avoid:

Abdominal Binders:
"Say NO to tight Abdominal Binders!"

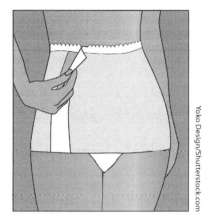

Yoko Design/Shutterstock.com

I advise all of the C-section postpartum moms I see for treatment to wear the elastic binder they got from the hospital for *only one or two weeks after surgery*. Ultimately I tell them to *say NO to abdominal binders* after that. They squeeze too hard and take over the work of the abdominal muscles, which will ultimately make them weaker. To flatten your postpartum tummy, you need to strengthen, not weaken your abdominals! Abdominal binders are not a quick fix to flatten your tummy, and in the long term they make that "Mommy Tummy" worse.

You may hear about these from celebrity moms or well-meaning "health and fitness professionals" who apparently lack a full understanding of how a woman's core muscles work. There are now a few companies and even a bestselling book that advises women to use tight abdominal binders to develop a flat tummy after childbirth. But I say STEER CLEAR.

*There may be some unusual circumstances where it is medically necessary to use an **elastic binder**,* like after a C-section. If you fall into this category, please discuss this information on binders with your healthcare professional. Don't buy or use a binder before you have this discussion.

Elastic Abdominal Bands

For now, say no to elastic abdominal bands. The elastic abdominal bands I found on the market were not made out of graduated compression material and many of them were too tight. So let me caution you: Even though these garments look much more comfortable, they can actually cause more harm than good.

Pelvic/Sacroiliac (SI) Belt:

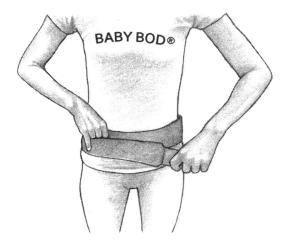

If you had a C-section, you can try using a Pelvic/SI Belt **after your stitches have been removed** and you can tolerate wearing the belt over your incision. Don't be surprised if it takes a few weeks to feel comfortable wearing the SI Belt.

This belt sits below the waist and wraps around your pelvic bones, and offers additional support to your unstable pelvis and weak core muscles. (After childbirth, the pelvis is often "unstable" and a Pelvic/SI Belt can be useful in preventing pain as well as improving overall function and wellbeing.) You can use it during your everyday activities or to give you extra support when you are trying to progress in your exercise program. Some women find it helpful to use when they sleep, or to prevent feeling pain when they roll over in bed or get up from bed. (**Note:** It can be used in conjunction with the compression shorts—wear the belt over the shorts —but it will not work over the **Baby Bod® Abdominal Wrap**.)

The Straight Leg Raise – Core Stability Test will help you determine if you are a good candidate for a Pelvic/SI Belt. (You'll find this test in Chapter Five; please follow the directions carefully.) Since you had a C-section, wait until after your six-week checkup and make sure that you have been given medical clearance to exercise before performing the test. If you want to try using the belt before your six week checkup, try one on and see if you feel like that support is helpful. (For more detailed instructions on Pelvic/SI Belts, please refer to *www.BabyBodBook.com.*)

Pelvic Floor Support Belts:

Pelvic Floor Support Belts are used to give an upward lift and support to the bottom of the pelvis. They can help with healing after childbirth by supporting the pelvic floor and allowing the soft tissue time to heal while in a supported position. If you had a C-section, you will need to wait until your stitches are removed and you can tolerate wearing the belt over your incision. These belts were originally designed to reduce the pain caused by varicose veins in the bottom of the pelvis, but they can also be used to control postpartum pain in the perineum. The upward lift should help reduce pain. Some women have told me that these belts also help to decrease the "falling out" feeling[E] they experienced right after childbirth because the belt helps to "lift the bottom of the pelvis upwards" and offers additional support to the pelvic organs.

You can start using a pelvic floor support belt one or two days after delivery, as long as it does not cause increased pain where you had a tear or episiotomy. To make the belt more comfortable, try placing a sanitary pad between your pelvic floor and the belt.

WHEN IS IT SAFE TO START EXERCISING AFTER A C-SECTION BIRTH?

It is perfectly safe and beneficial for most new moms to start a very gentle exercise program, like **Baby Bod**®, immediately after

---

[E] The "falling out feeling" is often a symptom of pelvic organ prolapse, which was discussed extensively in Chapter 7. If you do have this "feeling" please make sure to report it to your doctor or midwife.

a C-section birth. Most of you can start *most* of the **Preliminary Phase Exercises** the day after surgery. (The chart below will tell you which exercises are safe right after surgery, and which you should put off until it has been at least six weeks.) If you are groggy from taking pain medications or feel too sore from the surgery, wait a few days. Start them when you feel up to it. Go slowly, and follow each step as explained in the directions.

If you feel pain along the incision line, modify the exercise so you do not feel pain. If you cannot find a comfortable way to do the exercises during those first six weeks, stop doing that particular exercise and wait until you can do it without feeling pain. In the beginning, you may feel a little sore, but you may also find that doing the exercises relieves pain.

Here is a chart to make it easy:

Modified Preliminary Phase Exercises – C-Section Moms (First six weeks after surgery)	
What to Do...	**When to Start...**
Alignment Check	Only move the pelvis in pain free ranges when you do the *Alignment Check* and try to get into the neutral pelvis position and do the *Pelvic Rock Series*
Breathing Exercises	Do the *Lower Tummy Breathing* and the *Rib Expanders* as directed.
Pelvic Core Starter	Try to start the day after surgery. If you experience pain, use less force. If it continues to be painful, wait a day or two and try again.
Warm Ups	Start the *Head Bobble, Chin Tuck, Shoulder Rolls* and *Bali Dancers* the day after surgery. Wait until after your six-week checkup before starting the *Upper Back Stretch, Trunk Twister, Pelvic Rocks, Pelvic Circles* and *Pelvic Tilts*.
Walking Program	You can start the day after surgery as long as you have medical clearance from your healthcare provider.

When Should YOU Start?

If you had a *C-section within the last week,* you can start the *Modified Preliminary Phase* of exercises up until your six-week medical check-up. You'll find these exercises in Chapters Eleven to Fourteen.

If you are starting this program a *few weeks after you had your C-section,* but before your six-week checkup, do the **Preliminary Phase Exercises** up until your six-week checkup, and for at least one week before starting the more advanced stage of the **Baby Bod®** **Program.**

If you're starting this program *months after you had a C-section delivery,* do one week of the **Preliminary Phase Exercises** before progressing to the **Advanced Phase – Strengthening Exercises.** These will help you build a solid foundation for the more progressive exercises that follow.

What About Walking?

Initially, take two ten-minute walks a day and gradually build up to one thirty-minute walk a few times per week. On the days you cannot walk for thirty minutes, make sure to get in a few ten-minute walks.

For the first six weeks, I also want you to try your best to avoid inclines or uneven surfaces when you're walking outdoors. Then gradually return to walking on all surfaces after your six-week checkup.

When you are trying to return to certain activities, you may find a Pelvic/SI Belt useful in preventing pain in the pelvis and lower back. In fact, many moms find it especially helpful during the first several postpartum months when they use an elliptical machine or do any kind of workout that uses an incline or uneven surfaces. They find that it provides the additional support their body needs until they build up their core strength again.

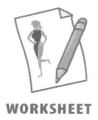

WORKSHEET

SIMPLE SELF-ASSESSMENT TESTS
Straight Leg Raise – Core Stability Test

If you had a C-section, **do not do this test until you are six weeks postpartum** and have been given medical clearance to exercise. The purpose to this self-test is twofold. It will help you learn how well your core muscles are stabilizing your torso and whether you would benefit from using a Pelvic/SI Belt.

Turn to Chapter Five to learn how to do the stability test, and record your results in the worksheet.

Diastasis Recti Test

This is a test to see if the connective tissue that lies in the space between your "six pack" abdominal muscles, the rectus abdominis, is taut enough to hold in your tummy. When the connective tissue is loose, it can cause an unsightly "Mommy Tummy."

Moms who had C-sections may do this test after they are six weeks postpartum and have been given medical clearance to exercise.

Please find the diastasis recti test in Chapter Seven.

Then record your results on the worksheet.

The Benefits of an Immediate Postpartum Visit with a Physical Therapist

I wrote **Baby Bod®** so that you, at the very least, would have a "virtual physical therapist" and evidence-based advice. But if you want ideal care, you'd do well to make an appointment with a physical therapist for a postpartum visit soon after you give birth.

It's not the norm to visit a physical therapist for a checkup within a week of giving birth, but it should be. This is the best way to ensure that your bones and muscles are aligned and working optimally so that healing can occur as quickly as nature intends. I have long encouraged my pregnant clients to come and see me for a postpartum checkup soon after they deliver their baby, hopefully within a week or so after the delivery. The ones who have taken my suggestion have typically enjoyed a smoother and quicker recovery.

During your postpartum checkup, your therapist might do a few manual therapy treatments, or see if you need additional support anywhere, such as the kind of support a Pelvic/SI Belt can provide. You will also be able to go over the **Baby Bod® Preliminary Exercises**, so be sure to bring your book and ask your therapist to check to see if you are doing the exercises correctly. Then it would be best to go back to your physical therapist after you are about six to eight weeks postpartum for a re-evaluation. At that time, you will be able to make a game plan for the most efficient recovery possible. If you are in pain, you may need to see your therapist a few times before the six to eight-week postpartum re-evaluation.

CONTINUED CARE OF YOUR INCISION

In the hospital, you will learn how to keep your incision clean and well moisturized, and how long to keep it bandaged. When you get the stiches or staples removed, ask your surgeon about any precautions that you need to take to encourage healing.

To improve the overall appearance of the scar, consider using silicone elastomer sheets. These can be easily found in your local drugstores or online. If your incision is fully healed, you can start using them as early as one month after you had the C-section. (You should discuss this with your surgeon, especially if you want to use them before your six-week checkup.) They should be worn twelve hours a day for approximately three months to be effective. (If you are nursing, however, you need to get medical clearance from your pediatrician prior to using them.)

DO SELF-MASSAGE TO SPEED HEALING

Self-massage is a simple way to help yourself feel better quickly. Any mom can benefit from the **Baby Bod®** self-massages below. Even if it has been months or years since you gave birth, you can still benefit from doing them. These massages can be used to ease the discomfort caused by common postpartum conditions such as constipation and diastasis recti, or pain in the abdomen, scar tissue and perineal area.[7, 8] You'll find these easy to do and very beneficial.

The massages I am going to give you are progressive. When you are doing any of the massages, *do not cause pain*. There may be some initial discomfort when you start, but do not press so hard that you cause pain or a burning sensation along the scar. In time, you will be able to progress by using deeper pressure, but only when you can tolerate it. Don't force it; more is not better.

Scar Tissue and Abdominal Massages

Scar tissue massage will help improve the mobility of the scar from the incision and prevent scar tissue adhesions from forming, which can eventually become painful. Massaging the abdomen will help speed up the healing process and improve the ability of the abdominal muscles to start working again. Moms who had

C-sections should not start doing Abdominal Massages until *after your six-week checkup and only if your doctor gives you medical clearance* to start massaging your tummy, especially the scar from your incision.

I am going to teach you three types of abdominal massages: The first one focuses on the scar tissue from the C-section incision and the abdomen; the second one is geared towards healing diastasis recti; and the last one is to prevent constipation. Make sure to start off by using gentle pressure; do NOT cause pain when you massage. Gradually build up the amount of pressure as you can tolerate it. Feel free to do these massages as you watch TV or listening to music.

Week One (After Six-Week Checkup)

Scar Tissue and Abdominal Massage

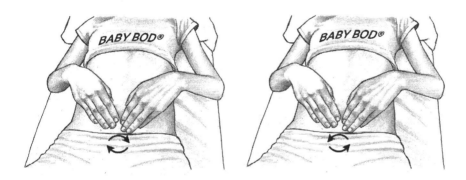

Scar Tissue & Abdominal Massage:
Use clockwise and counterclockwise strokes.

+ Place your two hands together and straighten your fingers. Gently press the pads of your fingers about 2 inches (5cm) above the scar.

+ Start on one side of the scar. (See illustration above.)

+ Press down lightly and start with very gentle circular strokes, first in a clockwise direction, and then in a counterclockwise direction. You should feel a gentle pull in your skin as you move your fingers in circular motions, but it should NOT be painful. (If you feel pain or a burning sensation along the scar, lighten the pressure until you don't feel either.)

+ Do this for two minutes.

+ Then move your fingers away from the start position to 2 inches (5cm) above the middle of the scar and repeat as above.

+ Then move your fingers again to the other side of the scar (2 inches or 5cm above) and continue massaging for about two minutes.

+ Massage a total of three areas above your belly button: one on the side, one in the middle and one area on the other side. Do this for a total of 6 minutes per day for one week and then progress to "Week Two to Four" below.

Diastasis Massage: Self-Massage for Diastasis Recti

Did you know that self-massage can help you heal diastasis recti? (Please refer to Chapter Seven to learn more about diastasis recti.) In my clinic, the women who do this massage often recover faster and are able to "activate" their core muscles more easily. If you had a C-section, you can start doing this massage *after your six-week checkup* if your healthcare provider assured you that your incision is well healed. (Yes, you can do this massage and the one above, and start them on the same day.)

Make sure not to press so hard that it causes pain. If you feel pain in specific spots, that is not so unusual. Just lighten up the pressure in the painful spots as you do the massage.

+ Place a flat hand on your tummy at the bottom of your ribcage. Press down gently to secure the skin as you do the massage with your other hand. (Refer to the illustration below.)

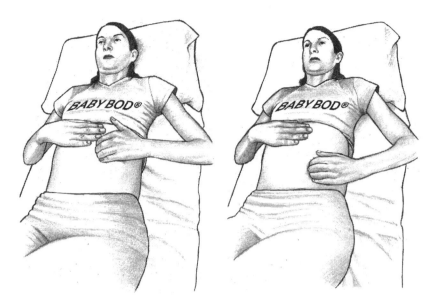

Diastasis Recti Masssage

+ Keep the fingers on your other hand together. Place your fingers about 3 inches (7-8cm) away from the midline of the abdomen. (Please refer to the illustration above). This hand will be massaging one side of the rectus abdominis muscle.

+ Gently press into the skin and maintain this pressure as you move your fingers downwards toward your panty line. It should feel as if you are *"pulling"* your skin downwards. You may even feel a slight burning sensation as you pull the skin, which is the effect you are going for. Although this is normal, do not press so hard that you cause pain beyond that slight burning sensation.

+ STOP JUST BEFORE THE SCAR FROM YOUR INCISION.

+ Do this about 10 times on each side of your tummy, every day, until your diastasis goes away.

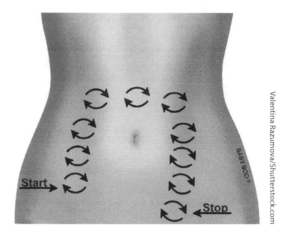

Constipation Massage Path

Constipation Massage[9]

The self-massage for constipation is simple and easy to perform. To do it, you'll use circular motions to work your fingers over a path of approximately ten spots in your lower abdomen. This will help move the bowel content. If you had a C-section, you need to wait until after your six-week checkup to give the incision time to heal.

+ Lie down in a comfortable spot like your bed. Place a pillow beneath your knees.

+ Place 2-3 fingers in the lower right side of your abdomen over the first massage spot, (please refer to the illustration above), and gently apply a constant and moderate pressure. If you experience pain, lighten up the pressure. Then maintain this pressure as you move your fingers in *clockwise circular motions* for approximately 10 seconds. (**Note:** Do not use counterclockwise strokes.)

+ Move to the next massage spot and repeat as above.

+ Gradually continue the clockwise massage circles up towards your rib cage, then across to the left side of your abdomen, and down to the inner-left side of your pelvis. Each massage path should last a total of one minute.

+ Repeat the entire massage path from your right side to your left side a few times, once a day.

Weeks Two to Four

Scar Tissue and Abdominal Massage

Continue the massage in all three areas on your tummy as you did during the first week, and add three additional spots. These will be *below* the incision. Each of the new massage spots should be directly below the three areas you started massaging during week one. There should be a total of six massage spots: three above the scar and three below the scar. As you progress, start to press a little bit harder, but not so hard that you cause pain. Alternate massaging clockwise and counterclockwise strokes for ONE minute in each spot. Massage a total of six minutes per day. Do this for one week and then progress by increasing the amount of pressure you use on a weekly basis until you reach Week Five.

Self-Massage for Diastasis Recti - Continue as directed above.
Constipation Massage – Continue as directed above

Weeks Five to Twelve

Scar Massage Circles and Abdominal Skin Rolling

Continue doing the Scar Massage (as above) for a total of three to four minutes. Then you are going to add "skin rolling."[F]

[F] Skin rolling can be very uncomfortable. If you find it painful, lighten up on your pressure by pulling less skin into the roll and don't press as hard with your fingers.

Abdominal Skin Rolling Massage

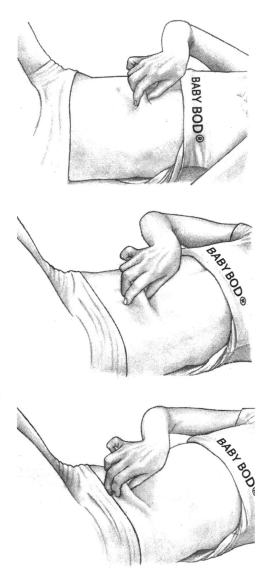

+ To roll your skin, gently grab a roll of skin in the upper part of your abdomen between your fingers and thumb.

+ Then move the "skin roll" down towards your panty line. To do this, use your thumb to push the "skin roll" towards your scar. Your fingers should "walk" towards your panty line as you push the roll with your thumb. *Stop just before you reach the scar.* Do not cause pain. (See illustration right.)

+ Do this along the middle of your tummy, then down the right side and then the left side.

+ Try to do this for 2 to 3 minutes after you do the massage circles.

Abdominal Skin Rolling Massage

Self-Massage for Diastasis Recti - Continue as directed above.
Constipation Massage - Continue as directed above.

Weeks Six to Twelve
Scar Massage and Abdominal Skin Rolling
Continue the same abdominal massage stokes as above, but this time you are going to *roll right over your scar* and continue until you reach the very bottom of your abdomen at your pubic bone. Stop if you feel pain or a burning sensation when rolling over your scar. Wait until you do not feel pain to include the scar rolling in your daily massage. Do as above for a total of five to six minutes.

Self-Massage for Diastasis Recti - Continue as directed above.
Constipation Massage - Continue as directed above.

Pelvic Floor Massage

Some women who have had C-sections have pain in their bottoms even if they were not able to deliver vaginally. Here is a massage you can do to relieve pelvic pain in the pelvic floor area. Please wait until after you had your six-week checkup before doing the pelvic floor massage.[7, 8]

Pelvic Floor Trigger Point Massage

This is a great way to relieve pain in the perineum, vagina and pelvic floor muscles. It might help make sex less painful too. Please wait until you are six-weeks postpartum before doing the trigger point massage. You can use an "S-shaped massage wand" or your finger to do a trigger point massage. (You can find one on our website or by Googling "pelvic floor massage wand.")

+ Use gentle finger pressure to find a spot that is painful in your perineum, the area between your vagina and anus or on the sides of your pelvic floor. You may also find painful spots inside your vagina.

+ Once you locate a painful spot (trigger point), gently press into the painful trigger point with your finger or the massage wand and hold it there for about 2 minutes.

BABY BOD® | 184

+ Make sure not to press too hard; it should feel as if you are causing the pain to increase a little, not a lot. As you continue to press, the pain should start to decrease. If the pain increases, either lighten up the amount you are pressing or skip that area and try it again in a day or two.

+ Then continue looking for more painful spots (trigger points). Press into the new trigger point for about 2 minutes and release (as above).

+ Try to alternate and press the trigger points at different angles when you repeat it the next day.

+ Try to do this on a daily basis until the pain and tenderness goes away.

    + **Note:** Instead of using your finger you can try this with an **"S-shaped" massage wand** that is designed for this purpose.

Self-Care Summary for C-Section Moms

Try to:

1. Avoid placing extra strain on your abdominal and pelvic floor muscles by **avoiding any movements that resemble a sit-up or crunch**. (Read more about the negative effects of sit-ups in Chapter Ten.)

2. Use a **pillow to support your tummy** when you move around and when you need to cough or sneeze, or while passing a bowel movement for a few weeks after surgery.

3. Reduce pain by applying "**iced gloves**" on your incision.

4. Get out of bed as soon as you have medical clearance and **walk** around a bit.

5. Prevent constipation by adding enough fiber to your diet and using **good toilet posture** (as discussed in Chapter Seven).

6. Use **external support** such as the **Baby Bod® Abdominal Wrap** or long-waisted medical-grade compression shorts to reduce pain and speed healing. Other helpful garments are the Pelvic/SI Belt and Pelvic Floor Support Belt.

7. Start the modified **Preliminary Phase** of the **Baby Bod® Program** a day or so after delivery, as laid out on the chart on page 156.

8. Use a **pillow to support the baby** when you nurse or bottle-feed your child.

9. Do the **abdominal self-massages** and pelvic floor massage after your six-week checkup.

10. Avoid **holding your breath** whenever you exert yourself.

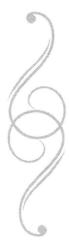

I hope these tips help and that you're starting to feel better. Go ahead and bask in the glow of your accomplishment and enjoy all those bonding moments with your new baby. Remember to be patient with yourself as you recover.

The **Preliminary Phase Exercises**, which span the next four chapters, should help. (Please remember to do the modified program). Just don't push too hard. Follow any special directions I give for moms who have had C-sections. Again, if you find any of the exercises painful, stop, and restart at a later date after you've had a chance to heal some more.

Just keep the faith…You *will* get that flat tummy back. In the meantime, stay off the scale. (See "Why the Scale Hasn't Budged Yet" in Chapter Two if you haven't already read it.)

Remember to be patient with yourself as you recover.

[1] Renfrew MJ, Lang S. Do cabbage leaves prevent breast engorgement? A randomized, controlled study. *Birth*. 1993; 20:2. doi: 10.1111/j.1523-536X.1993.tb00418.x.

[2] Roberts KL, Reiter M, Schuster D. A comparison of chilled and room temperature cabbage leaves in treating breast engorgement. *Journal of Human Lactation*. 1995; 11(3): 191-4. doi: 10.1177/089033449501100319.

[3] Annoni F, Pasche P, Torre R, De Stefano A, Annoni GA, Lucci C. Class 2 Compression Stockings According to ENC Standard with Innovative Features. *Minerva Cardioangiologica*. 2006; 54(3).

[4] Sawan S, Mugnai R, de Barros Lopes A, et al. Lower-Limb Lymphedema and Vulval Cancer: Feasibility of Prophylactic Compression Garments and Validation of Leg Volume Measurement. *Int J Gynecol Cancer*. December 2009; 19(9):1649-1654. doi: 10.1111/IGC.0b013e3181a8446a.

[5] Cheifetz O, Lucy SD, Overend TJ, Crowe J. The Effect of Abdominal Support on Functional Outcomes in Patients Following Major Abdominal Surgery: A Randomized Controlled Trial. *Physiotherapy Can*. 2010 Summer; 62(3):242–253. doi:10.3138/physio.62.3.242.

[6] Berman B, Perez OA, Konda S, et al. A Review of the Biologic Effects, Clinical Efficacy, and Safety of Silicone Elastomer Sheeting for Hypertrophic and Keloid Scar Treatment and Management. *Dermatologic Surgery*. November 2007; 33:11.

[7] Lewit K, Olsanske S. Clinical Importance of active scars: abnormal scars as and the cause of myofacial pain. *J Manipulative Physiol Ther*. 2004, 27(6): 399-402. http://www.eugenept.com/pdfs/clinicaimprtance.pdf

[8] Arung W, Meurisse M, Detry O. Pathophysiology and prevention of postoperative peritoneal adhesions. *World J Gastroenterol*. 2011; 17(41): 4545-4553. doi: 10.3748/wjg.v17.i41.4545.

[9] McClurg D, Lowe-Strong A. Does abdominal massage relieve constipation? *Nursing Times*. 2011; 107(12):20-22. http://www.nursingtimes.net/Journals/2013/01/18/m/y/j/290311Does-abdominal-massage-relieve-constipation.pdf

Exercise Guidelines

Congratulations! If you've made it this far, you know way more than the average mom about what it takes to bring about a full recovery and flatten that tummy! Now we're going to switch gears. In this chapter, we'll look at how to get the most out of the **Baby Bod®** **Exercise Program**. And then we'll get right to the instructions.

As I said before, there are two parts to the exercise program. No matter where you are on the birth continuum, you'll start with the **Preliminary Phase Exercises**—which you'll do daily along with a walking program. Then you'll graduate to the **Advanced Phase**—**Strengthening Exercises**, and continue on for six weeks. In that phase, we'll up the difficulty level of the exercises you already know and add about a dozen more. You only have to do these new exercises three times a week, but you can do them every day if you'd like.

TWO STAGES OF EXERCISES

In Chapter Six, I explained the rationale for the two-phase exercise program in depth. As I explained, the **Preliminary Phase Exercises** will re-train and "activate" your core muscles so they function cohesively as a group and work in proper coordination with your outer abdominal muscles. The exercises in this phase are so subtle they might not feel like "real" exercises at all—but trust me, they are necessary! Activating your core first will give you much better results from the strengthening exercises you'll add in the advanced program.

Working in this way will literally *strengthen your body from the inside out.* It will help you attain the right balance of strength between your core and outer muscles, and prevent you from developing *muscle imbalances* in your abdominal muscles. Your deeper abdominals will become stronger, even as you strengthen your "six pack" muscles—

Activating your core first will give you much better results from the strengthening exercises.

which is the RIGHT way to flatten that tummy.

If you're a fitness buff, you might be tempted to skip the first phase and go right to the advanced phase, or go back to your usual gym routine, before you are six weeks postpartum. Please don't. A little patience now—along with daily practice of the **Baby Bod®** exercises in right sequence—will bring you the fastest results overall.

Recovery is a step-by-step process. Because your body is in a different state, you can't just jump back into the same fitness routine you've always done. The point of the program is to provide you with exercise that is appropriate for you now, rather than give you exercise that's more than your body can currently handle. It doesn't make sense to put overstretched muscles—which need to be re-activated first—through a "boot camp"-style program in the first six weeks.

The best thing you can focus on right now is correcting your alignment (with the **Baby Bod® Alignment Check** in Chapter Eleven), reclaiming lost breathing capacity (with the breathing exercises in Chapter Twelve), warming up tight muscles (with the warm-ups in Chapter Thirteen), re-activating your core muscles (with the **Pelvic-Core Starter** in Chapter Fourteen), and getting gentle exercise with the walking program. I promise that you will get the fastest results if you do it this way.

A BRIEF OVERVIEW

What does the exercise part of **Baby Bod®** involve? How long will the program take to complete? That depends upon where you are on the continuum from pregnant woman to experienced mom:

+ If you are **pregnant**, start by doing the Preliminary Phase Exercises for at least one week prior to progressing to the six-week Advanced Baby Bod® Exercise Program.

+ If you are **newly postpartum**, do the Preliminary Phase Exercises until your six-week checkup, or for a minimum of one week, before starting the six-week Advanced Baby Bod® Exercise Program.

+ If you are an **experienced Mom and at least six-weeks postpartum**, start by doing the Preliminary Phase Exercises for one week prior to progressing to the six-week Advanced Baby Bod® Exercise program.

+ If you are **postpartum and have completed the initial six weeks of the strengthening program**, you can continue the Advanced Baby Bod® exercises as long as you like. I will provide you with even more advanced exercises in an upcoming sequel, *Baby Bod®: Get Your Core Off the Floor!* (Please keep an eye out for it.)

If an exercise isn't appropriate for you—given the kind of birth experience you've had—rest assured that I will mention that in the instructions for that exercise. (You'll also see general guidelines in the charts I provide.) Please pay attention to these; the information is there to keep you safe.

How to Progress with the Baby Bod® Program	
If you are Pregnant	Do the Preliminary Phase Exercises for at least one week prior to progressing to the six-week Advanced Strengthening Exercises.
If you are newly Postpartum	Do the Preliminary Phase Exercises until your six-week checkup, for a minimum of one week, before starting the six-week Advanced Strengthening Exercises.
If you are an Experienced Mom and at least six weeks postpartum	Start by doing the Preliminary Phase Exercises for one week prior to progressing to the six-week Advanced Strengthening Exercises.

Highlights of the Full Program

Walks
are important
if you want
good results.

- Do the **Preliminary Phase Exercises daily**. I'll show you how to do many of the exercises in different positions—such as lying down on a mat, sitting in a chair, or while standing or walking. This way, they're easier to "sneak" into your day in bits and pieces. It's actually better for you to do most of the exercises in this phase while going about your everyday activities. This will help you reprogram your body so everything works at optimal levels during ALL your normal daily activities, not just when you exercise. This is how to keep your **Baby Bod**® "ON" all day long. And by that, I mean, moving and using your body in the healthiest way possible, so you have plenty of energy to do what you need to do.

- **Add daily 30-minute walks**. These are important if you want good results. You can start with 5 to 10 minute mini-walks and gradually build up to daily 30-minute walks. And on the days you just can't manage a 30-minute walk, take three 10-minute walks.

- **At the appropriate time (see above), move on to the Advanced Exercises**. Continue the **Preliminary Phase** of exercises daily while adding these additional exercises three times per week. (If you're up to it, feel free to do them daily.)

- **If you'd like, add in a gym program**. Once you are able to start the Advanced Exercises, you can return to the gym. Do all the Preliminary Exercises first as a warm up and then do your strengthening exercises. Finish up by walking on the treadmill for 30 minutes or substitute some cardio equipment on the days you do not walk longer distances. Try to wait until you have completed at least 12 weeks of this program before adding weights such as cuff weights or the cable column, to your fitness program.

Do the best you can to stay on course and do your exercises daily, even in bits and pieces. If you miss a day here and there, you'll still get great results. If you have to skip more than a day, don't drop the program; return to it as soon as possible. On "off" days, make sure you use good alignment and good breathing techniques during your everyday activities, *which will help maintain core activation*—even if you can't exercise.

It May Be Common, but It's Not Normal to Pee When You Work Out

Recently there was a lot of discussion in social media and the news about how women female "extreme athletes" were proud that they lost urine while performing a deadlift. *This is not good.* Although this may be a common problem for women, it is not normal. And by that I mean that women's bodies are not designed to lose urine during daily activities. Leaking urine is a signal that something is wrong and that maybe because you are trying to do an activity that is too challenging for your current condition. If you experience this, this is what I advise: When you are doing an activity that causes you to lose urine, stop and try it again—this time making sure you are using good alignment (see **Baby Bod® Alignment Check** in Chapter Eleven) and exhaling while you exert yourself. If you continue to lose urine, try an easier activity, like carrying or lifting less weight. If that doesn't work, do this program and see if it helps. If not, go see a women's health physical therapist to resolve this problem.

HOW TO GET THE BEST RESULTS

1. **Follow the sequence provided for you in the Baby Bod® Program.**

2. **Use the right form.** Get your body in the best possible alignment

3. **Remember to breathe correctly.** Follow the instructions and count out loud as you exercise.

4. **Avoid exercises that are too challenging for your current condition,** no matter how tempted you may be.

5. **Don't "supplement" Baby Bod® exercises** with outside exercises that you think will speed your progress. Make sure to complete the **Preliminary Phase Program** and six weeks of the **Baby Bod® Advanced Program** before adding other exercises. If you push it too much, too soon, you could actually set yourself back.

Two Big Mistakes Mommies Make When They Try to Flatten Their Tummies...

Mistake #1 – Sit-ups:

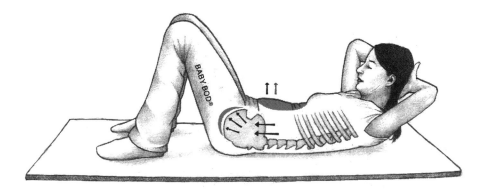

When you do a sit-up or an abdominal crunch, the pressure in your abdomen rises and places downward and outward pressure on your pelvic floor and lower abdominal area. Your pelvic floor and deeper abdominal muscles should contract strongly and automatically, like a trampoline, to match the increasing pressure. If your core muscles are not working optimally, *which is normal after childbirth*, the increased pressure will hone in on that area, and can cause the deep abdominal and pelvic floor muscles to become overstretched and weaker. So, you *run the risk of developing an unsightly "bulge" in the lower tummy and a droopy pelvic floor*. This can also lead to more serious problems, including problems like a leaky bladder, pelvic organ prolapse, and pain in the pelvis and lower back.

Here's yet another issue. Earlier in the book (in Chapter Seven), I explained how **diastasis recti** is caused by the spreading out of the *linea alba*, the connective tissue that runs down the middle of your abdomen. Guess what happens to this connective tissue when you do a sit-up? The increased pressure in your belly places further strain on the linea alba and causes it to spread out even more. This can increase the bulge some women develop in the middle of their tummies as a result of childbirth. This means your *"Mommy Tummy" can get worse, not better, if you do sit-ups.*

Does this mean you should never do sit-ups? The pelvic floor and your deep abdominal muscles are not normally trained to withstand the prolonged pressure created by *repetitive* crunches. *It's an endurance issue.* I personally prefer to teach women exercises such as those in Baby Bod® that flatten their tummies without increasing the pressure inside their bellies.

If you are unconvinced, and really want to do sit-ups or crunches, please do not do them unless you can do a sit up without your belly bulging. Try it. Lie on the floor and place a hand on your belly and do a sit up. If you did not feel your belly bulge upwards or your pelvic floor bulge downward, you may be able to do a few gentle sit-ups. But make sure to stop as soon as you feel your belly bulging.

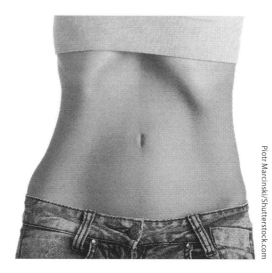

Piotr Marcinski/Shutterstock.com

Mistake # 2 – Pulling in Your Belly to Prevent Your Belly from Bulging

Yes, I know that many health and fitness professionals give this advice when they are trying to teach you to "turn on" your core muscles. They're well-meaning but misguided. I, too, used to give this advice before I fully understood how the different layers of abdominal muscles work in coordination with each other. Here's why you DON'T want to do this: Pulling your belly button towards your spine will encourage your outer "mover" muscles to take over the work of the deeper core stabilizing muscles. This can lead to weakening rather than strengthening the deeper abdominal muscles—the polar opposite of what core muscle exercises *should* do.

So if you are taking an exercise class or using an exercise video and the instructor tells you to "pull your belly button towards your spine to turn on your core muscles," DON'T. Instead, use good alignment and make sure to gently exhale to activate and "wake up" your core muscles.

IN SUMMARY

I hope you're excited about undertaking an innovative exercise program that will **strengthen you from the inside out**. Let's move on now to the first "exercise" in the **Preliminary Phase Program: the Baby Bod® Alignment Check.**

CHAPTER ELEVEN

Alignment – "How Do You Stack UP?"

Would you like to instantly look 5 to 7 pounds thinner?

Simply changing the way you carry your body as you move through your day can make you look five to seven pounds slimmer. This really is a great quick fix for your appearance while you're working on shedding that extra baby weight! But that's not all it does. As I said in the chapter on core muscles, when your bones and muscles are in the best alignment possible, your muscles—including the ones that hold in your tummy—work more efficiently.[1, 2, 3, 4, 5, 6, 7] They pull in your stomach more, which slims your profile.

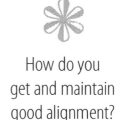

How do you get and maintain good alignment?

How do you get—and maintain—good alignment? That's what we're going to talk about in this chapter.

First, let's make the definition clear: When I say "alignment," I am speaking about how you stack your rib cage over your pelvis and your pelvis over your feet. (Please see "A Little Tweak, a BIG Difference," later on in this section).

A little further down, I am going to walk you through a simple, six-step series that will help you learn how to align and move your body in the most effective and efficient way possible. You NEED to learn this, because you'll use it as the "start" position for most of the exercises that follow. This will help you get your form right, which is essential for good results.

Here's the good news: Once you learn how to move with correct alignment throughout the day, you will activate your core muscles in the same way you would by doing the right exercises. Imagine that! And if you do this conscientiously with the other **Baby Bod®** **exercises**, you'll flatten that tummy in record time.

Why is it so hard for some people to change their alignment?

I bring this up because I see many postpartum moms for treatment in my clinic that have stiff and rigid areas in their torso and/or buttocks where muscles are in "clamp-down and hold" mode, and these rigid muscles prevent them from moving into good alignment. Normal muscles have the ability to contract and then elongate. Rigid muscles lose the ability to elongate. When this happens, there is a loss in flexibility, which leads to stiffness and pain and poor alignment habits. These can prevent you from getting rid of that "Mommy Tummy." If that's your problem and you want a flat tummy, you need to learn how to move through these areas *before* learning strengthening exercises. The **Baby Bod® Alignment Check**, in combination with the other exercises in the **Preliminary Phase Exercises**, will increase flexibility in these areas.

If you are pregnant now, please don't skip this chapter. Learning the **Baby Bod® Alignment Check** now will put you a step ahead in your recovery process. Realize, of course, that the bigger you get, the harder it will be to do this perfectly, especially when you try to align your ribcage over your growing belly. Just do the best you can. And be patient. After you have your baby, this will be much easier.

A Little Tweak, a BIG Difference

Look at the illustration below to see how much better you can look when you correct your alignment by stacking your rib cage over the pelvis. Which figure looks best to you?

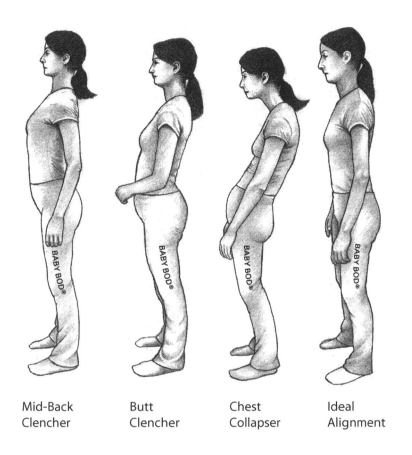

| Mid-Back Clencher | Butt Clencher | Chest Collapser | Ideal Alignment |

POSTURE VS. ALIGNMENT

Notice that I'm using the word "alignment" rather than "posture." I've chosen it for a reason. "Posture" is basically a snapshot of how you hold your body in a given moment in time. But the next moment, you move, it changes. "Alignment," however, is about how you *stack* your chest over your pelvis, and your pelvis over your legs, *as you move and rest* throughout the day. Posture is stationary and temporary. Alignment is dynamic, which means it changes as you move, even when you breathe! And since you are breathing and moving throughout the day, it's much better to focus on your alignment rather than static posture. I realize this might contradict what you always heard from your mom: "Fix your posture! Stand up straight and stick that chest out." She meant well, but as you will learn below, she was wrong.

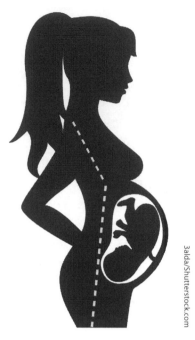

3alda/Shutterstock.com

Alignment Changes
The dotted line show how pregnant women tilt their chest up
and backwards to make room for the growing baby

ALIGNMENT CHANGES IN PREGNANT WOMEN

Before I teach you the Alignment Check, however, I want to help make you more aware of how you are carrying yourself now and how you may have developed dysfunctional alignment, especially while you were pregnant.

Alignment dysfunctions often develop when a woman is pregnant. Typically what happens is this: You move into the final trimester of pregnancy and your belly continues to expand to accommodate your growing baby. At some point, the baby becomes so big that the only way for the baby to grow is by pushing upwards against the diaphragm and outwards, as in the illustration above. As the area inside your abdomen starts to fill up, your upper body has to lift up and tilt backwards to make room for the baby! You learn to tilt backwards away from your belly to make more room for the baby.

As a result of these changes during your pregnancy, you needed a way to keep your balance and stay upright! How did you do it? You learned to "clench" muscles in your back and buttocks to hold that growing belly up against gravity. If you're like most women, you'll develop one or two "alignment adaptations" while pregnant to help counterbalance the size and weight of your pregnant tummy. Eventually, these areas become rigid and often become painful, which can lead to more serious problems down the road, such as a "Mommy Tummy," chronic pain and incontinence.

Post-Pregnancy Alignment Habits

When you're pregnant, you're just doing your best to keep your balance. But what happens if you *continue* to use these rigid alignment patterns even *after* you give birth to your baby? This is likely to happen because after childbirth, the abdominal muscles are stretched out and weak. This loss of support in the abdomen makes it harder to stand upright without clenching the muscles in your back and buttocks.

I see many very thin moms who come in to my practice for treatment and complain about pain, urine leakage or, their "Mommy Tummies" soon after giving birth—or even years after—and they're shocked when I point out that the way they move and carry themselves causes their bellies to bulge out, or causes the pain they are complaining about and/or incontinence. What they are doing is continuing to walk around as if they were still pregnant. They are using the same "clenching" or "holding" patterns they learned to hold up their swollen, pregnant bellies but never learned how to revert back to the way they carried themselves before they got pregnant. This can continue for years or even decades after childbirth!

A new client of my mine named Donna visited me with a decade long history of reoccurring lower back pain. She went for treatment with several different health care providers but nothing gave her permanent long lasting relief. Her prior treatment included advice on posture, core exercises and she even went for several spinal manipulations sessions; all resulting in minor temporary relief.

She was still carrying her body as if she was pregnant.

During our first appointment, I told Donna that even though it was over a decade since she had given birth, she was still carrying her body as if she was pregnant. I took a photo of her and used it to point out her alignment dysfunctions. As she looked at her own picture she was able to see how her rib cage and chest tilted upwards, which is often a tactic women learn during pregnancy to make room for their growing baby. Donna was really surprised to also learn that her back muscles developed a habit of "clenching" to help keep her chest and rib cage tilted upwards. These "clenched" muscles were preventing her from moving her rib cage over her pelvis. I explained to her that if she wanted to get rid of her back pain she needed to learn how relax her back muscles so that she would be *able* to improve her alignment and achieve longer lasting pain relief.

When I demonstrated how to restack her rib cage over her pelvis, Donna was able to do so easily by envisioning how her body behaved prior to pregnancy. She was able to actively "relax" her tight back muscles and realign her body. I took another picture of Donna and she was delighted with the way she looked. Donna returned for two more visits over the next month and reported that her pain was gone. She was especially delighted that her tummy looked flatter too.

I'll show you how you can change your alignment too, below, but first I would like to teach you how to identify and correct dysfunctional alignment adaptations that can cause you to clench muscles. Learning this will allow you to move with more fluidity and efficiency, and it will make you look thinner too!

Here is a list of the most common alignment dysfunctions postpartum women adopt. Which one sounds most like you? Or do you have a mixture of a few of them?

1. The Mid-Back Clencher (Military Posture)

In this dysfunctional holding pattern, the upper back is lifted up and tilts backwards, away from the pelvis. If you did this when you were pregnant, it's because you needed to make more room for the baby to grow in your abdomen. The size of the baby at the end of your pregnancy prevented you from being able to stack your rib cage over your pelvis.

In order to maintain this "tilted" position, the muscles in your mid-back have to work overtime by clenching in that area. This leads to developing a stiff and rigid area in your lower mid-back, which will prevent normal, efficient movement and increase the likelihood of developing back pain.

Can you guess another big problem with this alignment adaptation or clenching pattern?

Answer: Mid-back clenching behavior can prevent normal breathing patterns. The diaphragm cannot work at full capacity when the chest is held in the military position. The diaphragm, just like the other core muscles, works best when your ribcage is stacked over your pelvis and you use good alignment.

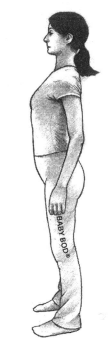

Mid-Back Clencher

2. The Butt Clencher

Pregnant women often develop this dysfunctional alignment adaptation to counterbalance the increasing weight in the front of their body by clenching the muscles in the buttocks tightly. Part of your pelvic floor (the posterior section) will also, almost certainly, be involved in the clenching. Your knees may also over-extend, curving backwards. Allowing this to become a habit can lead to knee degeneration and pain in the groin, hip, and the buttocks. Also, many women who are butt clenchers complain of urinary leakage, constipation and painful sex.

Are you a Mid-Back Clencher or a Butt Clencher? Or are you a mixture of both?[A]

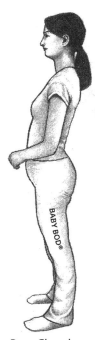

Butt Clencher

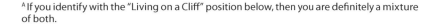

[A] If you identify with the "Living on a Cliff" position below, then you are definitely a mixture of both.

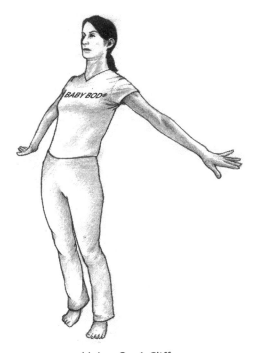

Living On A Cliff
This is a picture of a woman who is using "clenching behavior"
in both her buttock and mid back to stand upright.

3. Moms: Are You "Living on a Cliff"?

Some moms learn to use a mixture of mid-back and butt clenching behavior as a way to fight gravity. It causes them to stand in a way that I describe as "standing on the edge of a cliff." Here's what I mean by that. Try this:

+ Stand up on your toes, arch your back, and thrust your pelvis forward, as if you are standing on a cliff.

+ Try to keep your balance by holding your arms outwards, forming a cross. Imagine your arms are stretched out and clinging onto the walls of the imaginary cliff. You are "holding on for dear life!"

While you are trying this, I want you to think about what muscles you are clenching in order to maintain balance and prevent falling off the cliff. Right: your buttock and back muscles are clenched, with your chest pushed up high and knees smashed backwards. This clenching behavior can endure long after pregnancy.

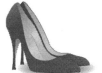

OCAL/Clker.com

What do you think happens to your body when you wear a pair of high heels? Wearing high heels can throw off your alignment and force you to clench the muscles in your back and buttocks. This, too, makes you feel like you are "Living on a Cliff."

4. Chest Collapser

Still other moms develop a habit of collapsing their ribcage downwards as a way to stand up against gravity. To counterbalance this position, the pelvis and neck are pushed forward and the buttocks are usually clenched. This can lead to neck, hip, pelvic pain and other dysfunctions. I often see women adopt this type of posture if they overdevelop their outer abdominal muscles by doing too many abdominal strengthening exercises at the expense of the core muscles, something I spoke about in detail in Chapter Six.

Does this feel familiar to you? Do you think you use any of these dysfunctional alignment adaptations to stand up against gravity? If you're not sure, I'll explain below how you can tell.

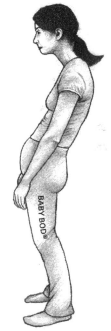

Chest Collasper

HOW TO IDENTIFY YOUR ALIGNMENT DYSFUNCTION

It's one thing to read about bad body alignment. It's another thing to identify yours. The best way to do that is to ask a friend, partner, mom or sister to take a side-view picture of you standing. Try to wear tight clothing or a bathing suit. It is REALLY important that you stand in your "normal" position, not the way you think you are meant to stand! You'll find that *pictures don't lie!*

Once you have the picture of yourself, please take a close look at the curves in your back and how you hold your body. What do you see? Compare your picture to the pictures above. Do you have any of these alignment dysfunctions?

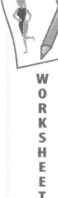

W O R K S H E E T

Do You Have Any Of These Alignment Dysfunctions?	
Mid-Back Clenching (Military Posture)	☐ Is your upper chest wall leaning backwards?
Butt Clenching	☐ Do you squeeze your buttocks tightly?
or Living on a Cliff	☐ Are you using a mix of both Mid-Back Clenching and Butt Clenching?
Chest Collapser	☐ Do you stand with your chest collapsed with your neck and pelvis pushed forward?

Record your findings on the worksheets and try to recheck your progress on a monthly basis.

If you identify with any of the above, it's worth the effort it will take to correct your alignment. Otherwise, as I said earlier, you could end up with aches and pains or problems like incontinence, soon, or even years after delivering your baby.[4] Leaning how to use your body differently may be frustrating in the beginning, but once you understand the concept and practice the **Baby Bod® Alignment Check**, it will become second nature. And you'll love how it will make you look!

How do you "stack up"?

Here's the easiest way to understand what good alignment is: Think of your body as having three different sections:

1. Your head, *chest and arms* are the top section

2. Your *abdomen, lower back and pelvis* are the mid-section

3. Your *legs and ankles* are the bottom section

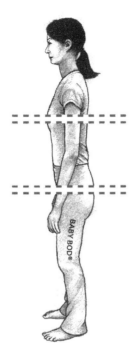

Your body works best when all three of these areas are stacked neatly on top of each other—when you are standing, sitting, or moving. This is what I call *ideal alignment*. Let me make it clear, however, that I do not want you to STAY in a static position, even if it is the "ideal alignment" position. You will learn what it feels like to be in this position and then try to maintain it as best as possible while moving during daily activities, sitting at your desk and while performing the **Baby Bod® exercises**.

It's important
to check
your alignment
several times
throughout the day.

HOW TO CHANGE YOUR ALIGNMENT BY REGAINING FLEXIBILITY: BABY BOD® ALIGNMENT CHECK

Let's talk now about how to move those tight muscles in the back, and sometimes the buttocks, that you clenched during pregnancy to hold your body up against gravity. **The Baby Bod® Alignment Check** will help you regain the flexibility that you lost during pregnancy even as it corrects your alignment. **Please do not skip this section**; it is the start position for most of the Baby Bod® exercises and it will help activate your core muscles.

Once you learn how to do all six parts of the Alignment Check, I'd like you to do it several times per day—ideally, once an hour or so. To make it easier for you to learn how to do this correctly, I am going to take you through a series of baby steps so you learn it bit by bit. This may give you the impression that the Alignment Check will take a LOT of time, but that's not true. Once you learn it, you can do it in a New York minute.

It is important to practice the **Baby Bod® Alignment Check** while *standing, sitting,* and *lying* on your back (while you exercise), so you can check your alignment throughout the day. (This way you can incorporate it whether you're sitting down and working on your computer or standing and waiting for water to boil, or when you are brushing your teeth, for instance.) In Chapter Seventeen, I will return to the Alignment Check and give you more advice on how to use it while moving through your day.

BABY BOD® ALIGNMENT CHECK:

Here's a brief summary of the **Baby Bod® Alignment Check** progression you will learn below:

- ✓ Neutral Pelvis Position
- ✓ Straighten Up Spine From Pelvis
- ✓ Exhale and Stack Chest Over Pelvis
- ✓ Shoulder Roll
- ✓ Chin Tuck
- ✓ Gentle Pelvic Floor Contraction

STEP ONE: NEUTRAL PELVIS POSITION

(**Note:** *If you had a C-section, only do this in pain free ranges. If you feel pain or pulling in your incision, decrease the range you are moving or wait until after your six-week checkup before doing this part of the Alignment Check.*)

The first step in correcting your alignment is to learn how to get your spine and pelvis back into the neutral position. "Neutral pelvis" refers to the midway point of your pelvis—where your pelvis isn't rotated too far back or tilted forward. This position is the key to good form when performing the **Baby Bod® exercises** and to correcting dysfunctional alignment, which leads to inefficient movement patterns.

Please take your time with this so you really get it down. Try to be patient with yourself in the beginning. You may find it very hard to tilt your pelvis in one of the directions, because the muscles are very tight in your back or hips. Don't force it. If you continue practicing rocking your pelvis in pain free ranges, the amount you are able to tilt your pelvis will naturally increase in a week or two. That is because you are allowing those tight muscles time to learn how to elongate again.

The first step in correcting your alignment is to learn how to get your spine and pelvis back into the neutral position.

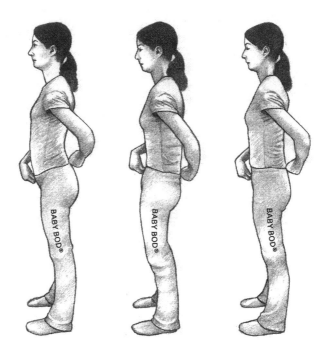

+ Stand with your knees slightly relaxed.

+ Place one hand on the front of your pelvis and the other on the back of your pelvis. Alternate rocking or tilting your pelvis forward and backwards *without lifting your chest*. Do this about 5 times.

+ **Stop** when you feel you are in between fully arching and fully rounding out your back.

+ *Try it in different positions*: Once you feel like you can get into the neutral pelvis position while **standing**, please practice it **sitting** and when you **lie down** on a mat to exercise. (If you are pregnant, do NOT do this while lying on your back; instead try it while lying on your side.)

+ **TIP:** When you try this in the *seated position*, **STOP** when you feel you are in between fully tilting your pelvis forward and backwards. Your pelvis should feel fully supported and stable on the chair. (Sometimes, my clients find it helpful when I tell them, "Stop when you feel like your vagina is resting on the seat of the chair.")

+ Next, go to Step Two: "Straighten up your spine from your pelvis."

STEP TWO: STRAIGHTEN UP YOUR SPINE FROM YOUR PELVIS

+ Stand with your knees slightly relaxed.

+ Maintain the neutral pelvis position and *let your spine rise up straight*, as if it is lifting up from the center of your pelvis. Pretend there are two helium balloons attached to the top of your ears pulling you upwards. As tempted as you may be, *do not raise your chest upwards*: That is the habit you are trying to break! (If you are having difficulty with this, refer to the sidebar, "An Easy Way to 'Straighten Your Spine'".)

+ ***Try it in different positions***: Once you feel like you can straighten up your spine while **standing**, please practice it **sitting** and when you **lie down** on a mat to exercise.

+ Next, go to Step Three, "Learn to how to stack your chest over your pelvis."

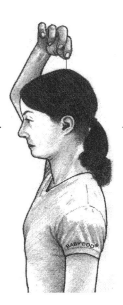

An Easy Way to "Straighten Your Spine"

Sit or stand in the neutral pelvis position and maintain that position as you gently pull ***one hair*** from the ***crown of your head***. Don't tug or pull it out! All you have to do is to gently pull upwards and imagine that it is pulling up your spine. You should feel as if your spine is being gently lifted through the middle of your pelvis. Got it?

STEP THREE: EXHALE AND STACK CHEST OVER PELVIS

Now that you know how to get your pelvis into the neutral position and how to straighten your spine, let's continue to learn the next step in the **Baby Bod® Alignment Check.**

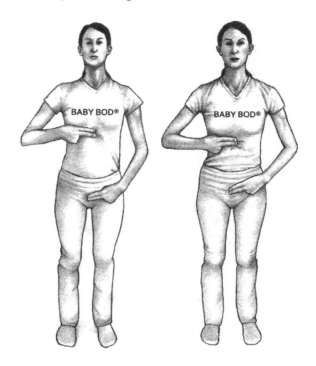

+ Stand with your knees slightly relaxed.

+ Progress by maintaining the neutral pelvis position with your spine rising up from your pelvis.

+ **Next, stack your chest over your pelvis:** Place two fingers on the bottom of the front part of your rib cage and place two fingers a couple of inches (5cm) below your belly button, right on top of your pubic bone. (Refer to the illustration above.)

+ Then *stack your chest over your pelvis* by GENTLY EXHALING as you move your chest downwards, towards your pelvis. You should see your two sets of fingers move towards each other, shortening the distance between your chest and pubic bone. (I like to tell my clients to "drop your nipple line without rounding out your upper back.")

+ *Try it in different positions*: Once you feel like you can stack your chest over your pelvis while you are **standing**, please practice it while **sitting** and when you **lie down** on a mat to exercise. Next, maintain this position and go to step four, "Roll your shoulders" to position them back above your ribcage.

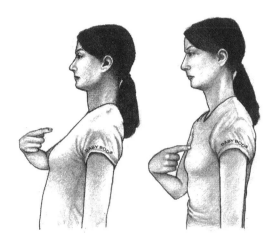

Are you having difficulty learning how to stack your chest over your pelvis?

Before you stack *your chest over your pelvis*, you may first need to learn what it feels like to move your chest forward.

Place one finger in front of your chest in line with the front of your pelvis. You may need to imagine drawing a straight line rising upward from the front of your pelvis. Keep your finger in that same position and move your chest towards your finger, as in the illustration above.

STEP FOUR: SHOULDER ROLL

A lot of moms have a tendency to develop rounded shoulders, especially after carrying and feeding a baby during the first few postpartum months. I am going to teach you how to get your shoulders positioned back where they belong, resting on the ribcage, not rolled forward.

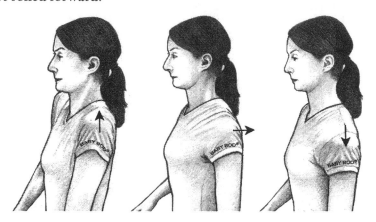

+ Stand with your knees slightly relaxed.

+ Continue to progress with the **Baby Bod® Alignment Check** by maintaining the neutral pelvis position, with your spine rising upwards and your chest stacked over your pelvis.

+ Then, *without moving your chest*, roll both of your shoulders up, then back, and let them gently drop down as in the illustration above. Don't force them. (Don't worry about rolling them forward; that is what you are trying to change.)

+ *You will have the tendency to raise your chest as you move your shoulders backwards: don't do it!*

+ *Try it in different positions*: Once you feel comfortable doing a shoulder roll while **standing**, try it while **sitting**, and while **lying down** on a mat.

+ Next, progress to Step Five, "Chin Tucks."

STEP FIVE: CHIN TUCK

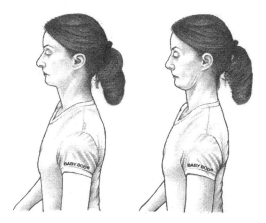

+ Stand with your knees slightly relaxed.

+ Progress while maintaining the positions in Steps One through Four.

+ Next, do a **chin tuck** *without lifting your chest upwards or bending your neck.* Try to keep your eyes looking straight ahead (pick an object in front of you to make this easier) and tuck your chin in and hold if for 2 to 3 counts. Then relax.

 Note: If you find yourself looking downward after you tuck your chin, you are doing it incorrectly. Keep your eyes looking at the same object straight in front of you throughout the entire time you hold the chin tuck.[B]

+ *Try it in different positions:* Once you feel comfortable doing a **chin tuck** sitting and standing, try it while lying down on a mat.

+ Next progress to one last step: Do a gentle pelvic floor contraction.

[B] This is something you can do to release neck tension while you are working on your computer or feeding your baby. It really does work to relax your neck!

STEP SIX: GENTLE PELVIC FLOOR CONTRACTION

+ The last step to the **Baby Bod® Alignment Check** is to maintain the Step One through Five positions and gently exhale as you do a gentle pelvic floor contraction, as if you are holding back one or two drops of urine (not a bucketful!). Hold it only for a second or two and then release.

Put It All Together

Practice the **Baby Bod® Alignment Check**. Do each step, one right after the other. Try to continue to exhale starting at Step Two through Step Six. That means you should slowly start to exhale as your stack your chest, and then continue while you roll your shoulders, do a chin tuck and then do a gentle pelvic floor contraction.

That's it!

Now go ahead and practice this entire series in different positions, while you're **lying down**, **sitting** and **standing up**. After practicing it and getting it down, it should only take a second or two to correct your alignment. As I said earlier, it is important to practice this because the Alignment Check will be the start position for most of the **Baby Bod® exercises**.

Let's review the steps one more time!

Baby Bod® Alignment Check:
✓ Neutral Pelvis Position
✓ Straighten Up Spine From Pelvis
✓ Exhale and Stack Chest Over Pelvis
✓ Shoulder Roll
✓ Chin Tuck
✓ Gentle Pelvic Floor Contraction

Once you practice this several times a day for a week or so, I think you will be able to do it automatically. Just be patient with yourself. Dropping bad habits and learning ideal alignment won't happen overnight. When you first learn, don't expect yourself to do it perfectly. Bit by bit, however, you'll find yourself moving more efficiently with more fluidity. That will happen faster, of course, if you take the time to do the Baby Bod® Alignment Check several times a day—ideally, once an hour.

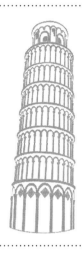

Do you feel like the Leaning Tower of Pisa?

When you do the **Baby Bod® Alignment Check** in the standing position, does it feel like you are leaning forward? Good! That is what you will feel initially until your body gets used to it and your eyes get used to looking at a new horizon line. It may actually take a week or two to get used to standing this way. Don't worry, your body will soon adapt to your new, improved alignment!

Baby Bod® Chest Alignment: Tape Trick

Are you having a hard time keeping your chest stacked over your pelvis, especially during your everyday activities? Or when you are doing the **Baby Bod® exercises?**

Here is a simple trick I used in my clinic for years. One of the simplest ways to make a permanent change in your alignment is to use tape as a portable biofeedback system. The tape will remind you when you are moving your chest out of alignment.

The type of tape I find most people can use without developing allergic reactions is *hypoallergenic medical paper tape*, instead of the tape used by athletes. You can find this type of tape in your local drugstore or online (you can check our store). Try to buy a brand that is at least 2 inches (5 cm) wide.[C] Another option is to take a look at the type of tape recommended in our website store *www.BabyBodBook.com.*

[C] If you're particularly allergy-prone, use a small piece of tape inside your forearm for 24 hours prior to using it to correct your alignment.

If you do feel itching or see a rash developing, remove the tape right away and clean the adhesive off your skin with rubbing alcohol on a cloth or pad. Then stop using it.

How to Use the Tape (Please refer to the illustration below.)

+ First, make sure to clean your skin thoroughly with rubbing alcohol or soap and water before you apply the tape. Then dry it thoroughly.

+ Next, measure the distance between the bottom of your rib cage to your panty line, and cut a piece of tape the same length. (You can use the tape to measure the distance by facing the sticky side out before you apply it to your abdomen.)

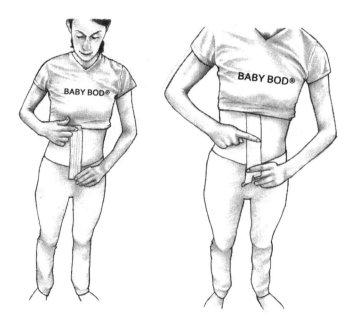

+ Before placing the tape on your tummy, do your **Baby Bod® Alignment Check** and *maintain that position as you apply the tape.* (This way, the tape will be taut enough so that you will feel when you tilt your chest backwards.)

+ Then apply the tape.

  + Place one end of the sticky side of the tape on the bottom of your lower rib cage. Press down and rub it upwards so that it anchors onto your skin.

  + Make sure to keep your chest positioned over your pelvis while you slowly press the sticky side of the tape along your belly until you get to just below your panty line.

+ Keep the tape on during the day, for no more than about 10 to 12 hours. Then remove it to give your skin a rest. Clean any adhesive residue off with rubbing alcohol on a cloth or pad and inspect your skin for any signs of an allergic reaction.

If this works well for you and you'd like to do this for a few weeks until you've learned to change your alignment, here's the best thing to do: Instead of running the tape down the middle of your belly, run it on either side of the belly button, alternating sides every other day. Continue to alternate the side you tape for the next four to five days. Then give your skin at least a day of rest before resuming use of the tape for another four to five days.

* * *

Congratulations! You just learned the first component of the **Baby Bod® Preliminary Phase Exercise Program**! Let's move on. In the next chapter, I'll teach you breathing exercises that will help relax you and also free up any restrictions in your breathing patterns that developed during the latter stage of pregnancy.

[1] Hodges PW, Sapsford R, Pengel LH. Postural and Respiratory Functions of the Pelvic Floor Muscles. *Neurology and Urodyamics.* 2007; 26(3):362-371. doi: 10.1002/nau.20232.

[2] Lee D, Lee LJ. Stress Urinary Incontinence- A Consequence of Failed Load Transfer Through the Pelvis? Presented at: 5th World Interdisciplinary Congress on Low Back and Pelvic Pain;November 2004; Melbourne,Austrailia. http://s3.amazonaws.com/xlsuite_production/assets/1436205/StressUrinaryIncontinence.pdf

[3] Sahrmann SA. *Diagnosis and Treatment of Movement Impairment Syndromes.* Arbor, Michigan:Mosby; 2001.

[4] Sapsford R. Rehabilitation of pelvic floor muscles utilizing trunk stabilization. *Manual Therapy.* 2004 Feb; 9(1):3-12.

[5] Hodges PW, Richardson CA. Inefficient muscular stabilization of the lumbar spine associated with low back pain. A motor control evaluation of transversus abdominis. *Spine* .1996; 21(22): 2640-50. http://www.udel.edu/PT/manal/spinecourse/Exercise/hodgesinefficientstab.pdf

[6] Carriere B. Interdependence of posture and the pelvic floor. *The pelvic floor.* New York: Georg Thieme Verlag; 2006; 68–8.

[7] Sapsford RR, Richardson CA, Maher CF, Hodges PW. Pelvic Floor Muscle Activity in Different Sitting Postures in Continent and Incontinent Women. *Arch Phys Med Rehabil.* 2008 Sep; 89(9):1741-7. doi: 10.1016/j.apmr.2008.01.029.

[8] Lee D, Lee LJ. *The Pelvic Girdle, an Integration of Clinical Expertise and Research, 4th Edition.* Churchill Livingstone: Elsevier; 2011

CHAPTER TWELVE

Let's Take a "Breather"

As you saw in the last chapter, pregnancy can really mess with your alignment. Now that I've helped you find the fix for that problem, let's tackle another one: your breathing.

Yup, pregnancy can mess with that, too.

As I mentioned earlier, there comes a point during pregnancy when the growing uterus pushes up against the diaphragm—one of your core muscles—and prevents it from descending when you breathe. The growing baby limits the normal excursion that is necessary to take in a deep breath. The bigger the baby gets inside the uterus, the more it blocks the normal movement of the diaphragm. As a result, the diaphragm can't move through its full range of motion, which means you aren't able to breathe to your full capacity. It also means that the diaphragm can't fully pull its weight as a member of the core muscle "team." Over time, the diaphragm can "forget" how to work at full capacity.

After you give birth, you can easily fix this. I've designed the **Baby Bod® Program** breathing exercises—which I will teach you below—expressly for this purpose. They are an integral part of its innovative and effective **Preliminary Phase Exercise Program**. The exercises are helpful whether you're still pregnant, you recently gave birth, or you had your baby quite a while ago and sense your body never fully recovered from pregnancy and labor.

Here's an added benefit: These breathing exercises are great at alleviating muscular tension or pain in the back, neck and pelvis. Just ten or fifteen minutes of these can make a huge difference, and once you learn them, you can do an extra set—beyond what I ask you to do as part of the program—any time you need quick pain relief.

Added Bonus: These breathing exercises can help relieve back, neck and pelvic pain.

LEARNING THE BREATHING SERIES

Postpartum Moms: You will be learning two different breathing exercises, the **Lower Tummy Breathing Exercise** and the **Rib Expanders**—each of which will help you reclaim full breathing capacity and the core stability you lost when you were pregnant. I would like you to practice these exercises in three different positions, supine (lying on your back), seated and standing.

Pregnant Women: You can do these exercises in three positions—lying on your side, seated and standing. It is best to skip the supine (lying on your back) position.[A]

When you exhale in these exercises, use very *little force*. Exhale as if you are cleaning a pair of sunglasses or as if you are trying to blow a cotton ball a few inches (8cm).[1,2]

Eventually, I would like you to try to incorporate these breathing exercises into your day—while you're feeding your baby, for instance, or waiting in line at the grocery store or sitting in the pediatrician's office. To make this easier on you, here's what I recommend:

1. Learn the breathing exercises while lying on your back first, unless you are pregnant. If you are pregnant, learn them while lying on your side first. Practice them for three to five minutes each, twice a day for a week. (If you're using them for pain relief, however, keep going for ten to fifteen minutes.)

2. Learn them in the seated position the following week. Practice them for three to five minutes each twice a day. During the second week you can do additional ones when you lie down to rest or if you feed your baby while in the side-lying position.

3. Then during the third week, learn them in the standing position and practice them for three to five minutes each twice a day.

[A] The Committee on Obstetric Practice of the American Congress of Obstetricians and Gynecologists (2009) recommends that pregnant women stop exercising in the supine position after the first trimester. To play things safe, try to avoid exercising while in the supine position throughout your pregnancy, that way you will not need to remember when to stop after the first trimester.

Once you're comfortable, you can do the exercises while standing, try doing the exercises in each of these three positions once a day for a minute or two in each position. You can do them at different times of the day to make it easier to fit into your schedule.

Note: If you skipped Chapter Eleven, go back and learn how to do the **Baby Bod® Alignment Check** before doing the breathing exercises. You will need to get into good alignment prior to doing each of the breathing exercises.

LOWER TUMMY BREATHING EXERCISES: B

1. Elevated Lower Tummy Breathing – Supine Position (Pregnant women must do this exercise in the side-lying position. For instructions, see below.)

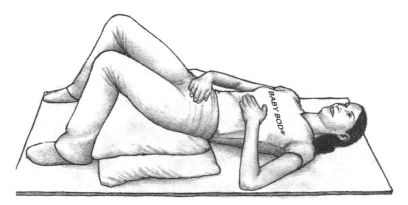

+ Do a **Baby Bod® Alignment Check.**

+ Then place one hand on the top of the lower part of your rib cage so that the upper part of that hand is resting on your ribs and the lower part of your hand is resting on your upper abdominal muscles.

B Bonus: This is a particularly good exercise to use to help release tension or pain in the mid or lower back, neck, or pelvis, especially in the supine and side lying positions. Again, if you use it for that purpose, stretch it out for 10 to 15 minutes.

- Place your other hand just above your pubic symphysis or pubic bone. This is the bone that lies a few inches (about 8cm) below your belly button and just above your lady parts. (See the illustrations above.)

- Pretend there is an inflexible tube made of hard plastic that starts at your throat and runs down towards your pubic symphysis. At the end of the tube, just under your lower hand, is an imaginary semi-inflated balloon the size of a pair of rolled up socks.

- Imagine that you are going to use this tube to breathe through, so that *when you inhale, you do not raise your chest.*

- Keeping this image in mind, *take in **short, shallow breaths** and **gently exhale*** (as if you are cleaning a pair of sunglasses), so that the air can cause a slight inflation and deflation of your imaginary balloon.[c] Use your lower hand to feel this motion in your lower tummy.

- While breathing, try not to move your chest. Monitor this with the hand you have placed on the border of your ribs (where the upper tummy meets your lower rib cage).

- Do this exercise for three to five minutes twice a day for a week, then progress to trying it in the seated position.

Tip: Try to use this exercise before falling to sleep at night or, if you are a smart new mom, just before you try to take a nap during the day.

---

[c] This is not meant to be a deep breathing exercise. Don't try to take in big breaths. Use shallow breaths and try not to forcibly expand your belly when you do this exercise.

Elevated Lower Tummy Breathing – Side-Lying Position (Good for Pregnant Women)

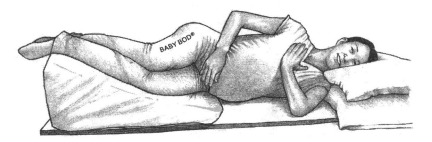

+ If you are pregnant, skip the supine position and do this instead: Lie on your side, elevate your pelvis above chest level with a pillow wedge or a few pillows, and follow the directions above.

+ Depending upon the size of your belly, you may find it difficult to feel your lower tummy slightly inflate and deflate under your hands. Please try it out anyway; it will make it easier for you to do after you deliver your baby.

+ Do this exercise for three to five minutes twice a day for a week, then progress to trying it in the seated position.

2. Lower Tummy Breathing Exercise – Seated Position

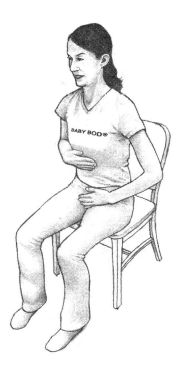

+ Now try this while seated. Begin by sitting and doing your Alignment Check. Then follow the directions above. Do this exercise for three to five minutes twice a day for a week, then progress to trying it in the standing position

Tip: Once you get the hang of this, you will be able to do it without holding your hands against your body. Try to do the lower tummy breathing exercise while performing normal everyday activities, such as feeding your baby or working on a computer.

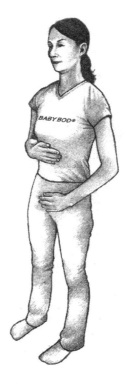

3. Lower Tummy Breathing Exercise – Standing Position

* Now try this while standing. Begin by standing and doing your Alignment Check, then follow the same sequence you did while doing this exercise in the supine and seated position. Do this exercise for three to five minutes twice a day.

Tip: Once you are able to do this without using your hands to monitor movement, try to do the lower tummy breathing during the day, like when you are cooking, talking on the phone, or waiting on line to pay for groceries.

After the third week, try to do the lower tummy breathing exercise in each of these three positions for a minute or two each, either all at once, or if it's easier, by sneaking in a few mini sessions throughout the day.

That's it for the lower tummy breathing exercises. Now let's learn an exercise that will further improve your breathing patterns: the Rib Expanders.

RIB EXPANDERS

You will need to use an old tie or a large scarf when you first learn this exercise. The purpose of the exercise is to help you relearn what it feels like when your ribs expand laterally or sideways.

Rib Expanders Supine – With Old Tie (NOT for pregnant women)

(**Note: Pregnant women can** start the rib expander exercise in the seated position and then progress to the standing position.)

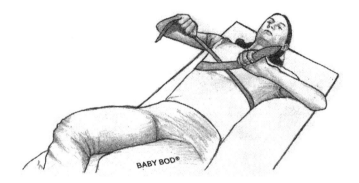

+ Lie on your back with your knees bent.

+ Do a **Baby Bod® Alignment Check.**

+ Place an old tie (or a long scarf) around your lower rib cage and crisscross the ends. Hold the ends of the tie in front of your body with both hands. (Please refer to illustration above.)

+ Gently pull the ends of the tie in opposite diagonal directions so that it slightly tightens around the rib cage.

+ Next, inhale and let the tie expand with your ribs by releasing your hold on the tie as you breathe in. (Release a little pressure: just enough so your rib cage expands, but not so much that the tie feels loose around your rib cage. It should always feel slightly tight around your rib cage throughout the exercise.) Feel your rib cage expand laterally (sideways) against the tie.

+ Softly exhale and gently tighten the tie as your lungs deflate and the rib cage relaxes. Let the tie follow the movement as your ribs return to their original position.

+ Just before you take in another breath, help your rib cage remember how to expand by using the tie to do an inward press and release: pull the ends of the tie so that they gently press your ribs inwards and then quickly release it.

+ Inhale and release the pressure, letting the tie follow the movement of your rib cage.

+ Exhale and tighten the tie as your lungs deflate.

+ Do another quick inward press and release.

+ Inhale again.

+ Exhale again.

+ Do another quick inward press and release.

Continue this for exercise two to three minutes twice a day in the supine position for one week, and then progress to the seated position. (Please see below.)

Tip: Now that you have the hang of how the rib cage should expand when you inhale, *try your best NOT to involve your belly muscles.* The point of this exercise isn't to take a deep abdominal breath and watch your belly expand. Your focus is helping your ribs remember how to expand laterally (sideways) as fully as they're meant to do during inhalation.

Tip: *Focus on keeping your rib cage down throughout this exercise.* The natural tendency is to tilt your rib cage up towards the ceiling when you inhale, but don't. Keep your rib cage aligned over your pelvis throughout the entire exercise.

Rib Expanders – Seated Position
(OK for pregnant women)

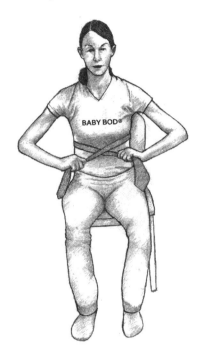

If you are *postpartum*, after doing the Rib Expanders for one week in the supine position, try this while sitting on a chair. If you are *pregnant*, you will have to start the Rib Expander exercise in the seated position.

Begin by sitting and doing your Alignment Check. Then follow the directions above. Do this exercise for two to three minutes twice a day for a week. Once you feel that you can do this exercise in the seated position, progress to trying it without using a tie. After that you can progress to trying it in the standing position.

Rib Expanders – Standing (OK for pregnant women)

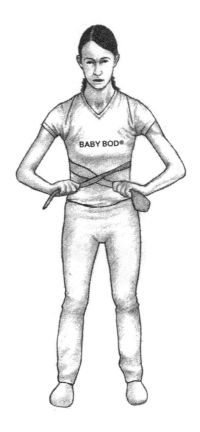

Both postpartum moms and pregnant women can progress to doing the Rib Expanders in the standing position after they have practiced it in the seated position for one week.

Begin by standing and doing your Alignment Check. Then follow the directions above. Do this exercise for two to three minutes twice a day for a week. After practicing the Rib Expanders standing with a tie, try it without using a tie.

After practicing this for one week, progress to doing the Rib Expanders in *all three* positions if you are *postpartum*, or *two positions* if you are *pregnant*. Do them for a minute or two each, all at once if you can. If not, fit them into a few mini-sessions throughout the day.

Rib Expanders – Without An Old Tie

+ Once you feel you can do this exercise successfully with the old tie, you can try it without using the tie. Instead, **use your hands against your rib cage.** First try it in the supine position, then while sitting and standing. (Note: Skip the supine position if you are pregnant.) Place your hands on the sides of your rib cage and do the exercises as explained above. Let your hands gently press your rib cage as you exhale, and release the pressure as you inhale. (Refer to the illustration below.)

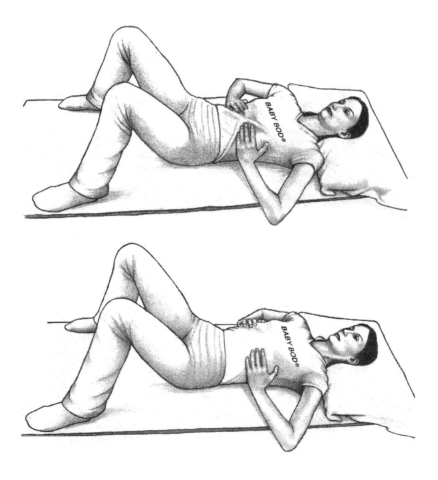

* * *

That's it for the breathing exercises. Let's move onto the next chapter and learn some warm-up exercises you'll use every day.

[1] Kitani LJ, Apte GG, Dedrick GS, Sizer PS, Brismee JM. Effect of Variations in Forced Expiration Effort on Pelvic Floor Activation in Asymptomatic Women. *Journal of Women's Health Physical Therapy*. January/April 2014; 38(1):19-27.doi: 10.1097/JWH.0000000000000005

[2] Hodges PW, Sapsford R, Pengel LH. Postural and Respiratory Functions of the Pelvic Floor Muscles. *Neurology and Urodyamics*. 2007; 26(3):362-371. doi: 10.1002/nau.20232

CHAPTER THIRTEEN

Warm Ups and Walking

In this chapter, I'm going to teach you some gentle warm-up exercises. These warm ups are so safe you can even do them while you're pregnant and begin them again the day after you give birth—with a few exceptions. If a particular exercise isn't right for you given the kind of birth experience you had, I will clearly indicate that in the instructions for that exercise.

Ideally, you'll do these daily. If you can only manage to do these a few times a week, however, go ahead—you'll still get great benefits from doing them. Many women, for instance, find that the exercises reduce the aches and pains that can occur when you're postpartum. Make time to learn them and then, once you've learned, try to squeeze them in when you are doing other everyday activities like feeding your baby, waiting for the water to boil in your kitchen, or watching TV. This is what my clients have done and it worked for them!

Yes, you can do this! You can bite off little pieces during the day, if that's easier. You also have the option of doing the entire series in one stretch.

Many women find that the exercises reduce the aches and pains that can occur when you're postpartum.

Ideally, you'll do these warm ups and walking daily.

Neck Stretches

1. Head Bobble: To begin, sit or stand in good alignment.

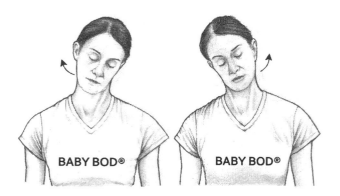

+   Bend the upper part of your head to each side. You should feel as if you are gliding your jaw sideways. This is different than dropping your ear towards your shoulder. (If you are bending your head towards the right, you should feel a stretch in the muscles just below your left ear.)

+   Do this 5 times to each side.

2. Chin Tuck: To begin, sit or stand in good alignment.

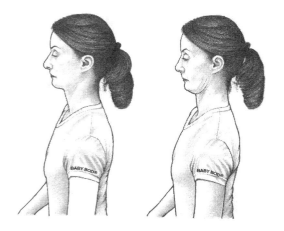

+ As you keep your eyes looking straight ahead, tuck your chin in and hold for 2 or 3 counts. Then relax. (If you find yourself looking down after you tuck in your chin, you are doing it wrong. Keep your eyes looking at the same object throughout the entire stretch.)

+ Repeat 5 times.

3. Shoulder Rolls: To begin, sit or stand in good alignment.

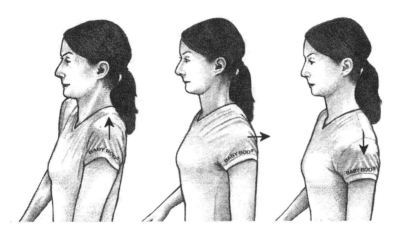

+ Without moving your chest, move your shoulders up, back and down.

+ Do this 5 times.

4. Upper Back Stretch: To begin, sit on a chair and place a 4-inch foam roll or a towel roll between your mid-back and the chair back. (**Note:** *If you had a C-section, wait until your doctor gives you medical clearance to exercise at your six-week check-up before doing this exercise*).

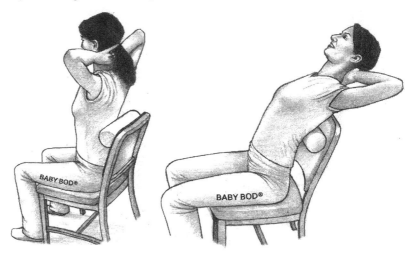

+ Raise your arms and place your hands behind your neck.

+ Gently lean against the foam roll (or a towel roll) and arch backwards. You should feel the stretch in your upper back.

+ Do this 5 times.

5. Bali Dancer: To begin, stand in front of a mirror, and get into good alignment.

+ Keep your shoulders level at all times. You'll notice a tendency to shrug your shoulder, so place the opposite hand on the shoulder you are exercising and hold it down. I will explain how to do this on the right side of your body; once you've done that, please also do this on the left side of your body.

+ Looking straight ahead, bend your right elbow and wrist as if you are a waiter carrying a tray in a restaurant.

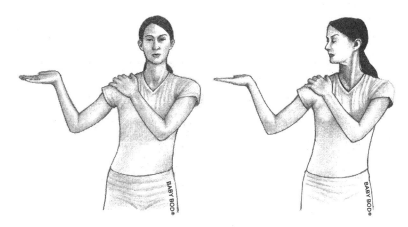

+ Place your left hand on your right shoulder and use it to hold your shoulder down during the exercise.

+ Then turn your head towards your shoulder.

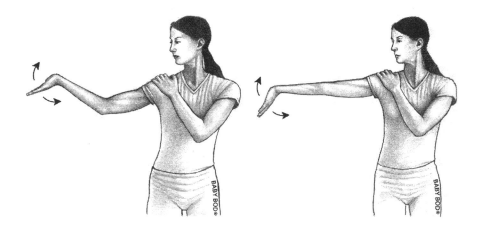

+ Keep your wrist bent and try to SLOWLY straighten out your elbow without shrugging your shoulder. Stop just before the point that you feel "tightness" in your arm (usually around your elbow), discomfort, pain, or tingling. This means that you may need to do the exercise with your elbow slightly bent.

+ Stay in that position and move your wrist up and down 10 times. (*continues next page*)

+ Repeat this two times a day on both sides of your body until you are able to straighten out your elbow and have your wrist bend up and down without any feeling tightness around your elbow or discomfort like the picture below.

6. Trunk Twister: To begin, lie on your back with one knee bent and your foot on top of the other leg. (**Note:** *If you had a C-section, wait until your doctor gives you medical clearance to exercise at your six-week check-up before doing this exercise*).

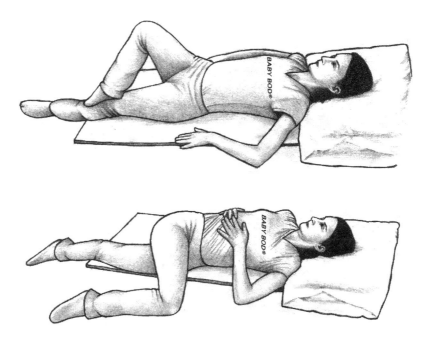

+ Place your hands on your tummy and then drop your bent knee towards the opposite side until the bent knee touches the mat.

+ Do this 2 to 3 times to each side.

7. Pelvic Rock Series

(**Note:** *If you had a C-section, wait until your doctor gives you medical clearance to exercise at your six-week check-up before doing these exercises).*

Make sure to move in pain-free ranges only. If one side lifts higher than the other, don't force it—just move within a range that makes you feel good. You many notice that the amount that you are able to move may increase after doing these warm-up exercises for a week or two.

7a. Pelvic Up and Downs: To begin, stand in front of a mirror with your knees relaxed. Get into good alignment.

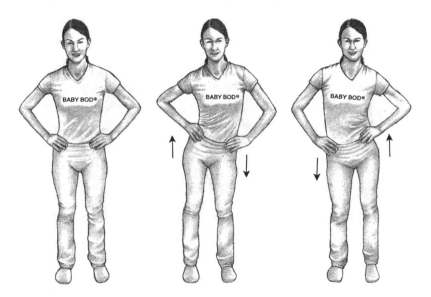

+ Place your hands on both sides of your pelvis.

+ Lift one side of your pelvis up toward the ceiling while the other side of your pelvis moves down toward the floor. Then reverse.

+ Do 5 times in each direction.

7b. Pelvic Circles: To begin, stand in front of a mirror with your knees relaxed. Get into good alignment.

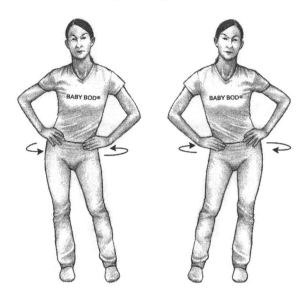

+ Place your hands on both sides of your pelvis.

+ Move your pelvis in a circle to the right 5 times then the left 5 times.

+ Do not force your pelvis to move into painful ranges.

7c. Pelvic Tilts: To begin, stand in good alignment with your knees relaxed.

+ Place one hand in front of your pelvis and the other hand in back of your pelvis. (Please refer to the illustration below.)

+ Tilt your pelvis forward and backwards by arching your lower back and rounding it out several times.

+ Keep your upper chest and shoulders still. You should feel as

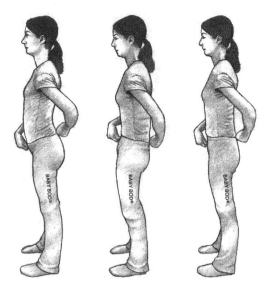

if you're pivoting your pelvis forwards and backwards while your upper chest and shoulders remain static.

+ Do this 5 times each way.

Great! You've just learned the warm-up exercises I'd like you to try to do every day.

WALKING PROGRAM:

The other thing I'd like you to add is a *daily walking program*. Walking is one of the easiest exercises for new moms and you can do it with or without your baby. During the first few months, try to use a stroller rather than a front carrier if you are walking longer distances or for more than ten minutes at a time.

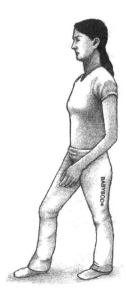

Depending on how you feel and if you have medial clearance to get out of bed, you can start walking very soon after delivery. I am not talking a marathon! Just try to move around as soon as you get the OK from your midwife or doctor. I am living proof that you can start walking almost right after delivery! Something happened to my brain right after I delivered my first daughter; it was back in the days where you had to lie down on your back to deliver. After I passed the placenta, I hopped off the table and started to walk out of the delivery room. Since they had taken my baby to the nursery, I didn't think there was any reason to stick around in that sterile room. The doctor had to yell at me to get back on the table because she had to stitch me up! She also mentioned she had never seen a woman do that before...I think I just wanted to naturally walk the pain off.

Try to take at least two ten-minute walks per day.

Try to take at least **two** ten-minute walks per day and gradually build up to one thirty-minute session of walking per day. First, start out walking around your room or the hospital hallways for a few minutes at a time, and then build it up to two ten-minute walks. Gradually increase the time you walk to thirty minutes a day or at least a few times per week. On the days you can't get in a thirty-minute walk, make sure to get in your ten-minute walks. For the first six weeks, try to stay away from walking on hills or inclines.

If you are taking the baby, try not to use a front carrier when you are walking longer distances. Use the stroller instead. When you use the stroller, try to choose routes that keep you on level surfaces for the first few weeks. Please do not carry the stroller down a flight of stairs, or lift it into a car for at least six weeks after childbirth. Until you have gone through the initial stage of healing, you should NOT carry anything heavier than your newborn baby.

If you're going for a walk by yourself or with a friend or family member, try not to carry anything! And if you have to carry something, make sure that it weighs no more than a few pounds. If you are in the habit of carrying a pocketbook, weigh it—you might be shocked! If it's more than a few pounds, take out the nonessentials.

* * *

Let's move on to the next chapter, where I will take you through a series of mini lessons that will help prepare you for the Pelvic-Core Starter, an absolute miracle-worker of an exercise. When you do this exercise correctly, you'll LOVE the results!

CHAPTER FOURTEEN

The Pelvic-Core Starter
The Final Pieces of the Baby Bod®
Preliminary Phase

Okay, you're ready for the *Pelvic-Core Starter*! This special exercise will do *miraculous* things for your lady parts. (Can you say *"Ooh la la"*?) It will help make sex yummy again!

Earlier, in Chapter Six, I explained one unfortunate consequence of pregnancy and the birthing process: The core muscles "forget" how to work, especially in coordination with the other abdominal muscles. Well, the Pelvic-Core Starter is a superstar here because it uses a mix of slow contractions and quick flicks to "wake up" different kinds of muscle fibers. That's why I named it the "Pelvic-Core Starter"; it's so good at strengthening the pelvic floor and deep abdominal muscles.

In fact, it's far superior to Kegel exercises, which isolate the pelvic floor muscles. Traditional Kegel exercises do not take into account the fact that the pelvic floor muscles are part of the core muscle system, which means these muscles work best when you use correct breathing techniques AND align your body, as you do with the **Baby Bod® Alignment Check**. The Pelvic-Core Starter gets all your core muscles working together, as nature intends. If you do it conscientiously, it will help give your body the firm foundation it needs so it can once again be strong, healthy, and sexy.

In this chapter, I want to teach you how to feel a pelvic floor contraction and then, once you've mastered that, how to do the Pelvic-Core Starter exercise.

The Pelvic-Core Starter gets all your core muscles working together, as nature intends.

THE RIGHT WAY TO CREATE A PELVIC FLOOR MUSCLE CONTRACTION

Before you jump ahead and try to do the Pelvic-Core Starter exercises, I want to make sure you really know how to *correctly* contract your pelvic floor muscles.

OK, I can hear you… "Isn't that a Kegel exercise? We all know how to do Kegels! My doctor gave me a piece of paper that explained how to do them. Heck, there must be thousands of articles telling you how to do them. Of course I know how to do a Kegel. Gosh!"

Stop right there!

Do you know many women who think they know how to contract their pelvic floors do it incorrectly? Studies have shown that a large percentage of women hold their breath or even push downwards as they attempt to do a pelvic floor contraction.[1] If you do a pelvic floor contraction properly, it should feel as if you are "lifting" your "lady parts" upwards, not downwards. I would like you to go through the following lessons to learn how to feel for a correct pelvic floor contraction and to make sure you are not working against your recovery.

Creating a Pelvic Floor Muscle Contraction with Finger Palpation

You may try this method if—and ONLY if—your health care provider did **not** tell you to avoid sex or to avoid inserting anything in your vagina. Most moms must wait until after their six-week postpartum checkup prior to using this method to feel a pelvic floor contraction. You may also try this if you are pregnant and have not been given any restrictions from your doctor or midwife. (If you have long nails, you might want to cut them first.) (**Precaution**: If you had a Grade 3 or 4 tear, start after six-week check up.)

The best place to try this is while you are sitting on a toilet or the edge of your bed. To do this:

+   Insert a *clean* finger inside your vagina, just about 2 inches (5cm).

+ EXHALE gently and try to tighten your vagina around your finger by imagining that you are trying to stop the flow of a *few drops* of urine.

+ You should feel the muscles gently tighten around your finger. As you get stronger, you will feel as if your finger is being pulled upwards towards your chest.

+ Hold it for 3 seconds and then relax.

+ Once you are able to feel the pelvic floor muscles contract, try to feel them relax. It should feel as if the muscles melt a bit. There should be less tension around your finger when the pelvic floor muscles relax.

How to Feel a Pelvic Floor Muscle Contraction (Without Finger Palpation)

Right after childbirth, your doctor or midwife will instruct you to avoid inserting anything into your vagina (such as a tampon or a penis) until you make it through your six-week postpartum checkup. Here are two different ways you can feel a pelvic floor contraction without inserting a finger. This is also appropriate for pregnant women or other women who have been instructed not to insert anything in their vaginas. If you were not given these restrictions, you may also try this method to make sure you know what it *feels* like when you contract your pelvic floor muscles. (**Precaution:** If you had a Grade 3 or 4 tear, start after six-week check up.)

Method One:

+ While you're urinating, EXHALE gently and try to stop the flow of urine *midstream* and feel the muscles contract as you hold back your urine.

+ Do this ONLY for a few seconds; then continue to urinate and empty your bladder.

Make a mental note of how it feels to contract your pelvic floor muscles and how it felt when you relaxed your muscles to continue urinating.

CAUTION: To prevent developing urinary tract infections, never do this more than once a week. Do not use this method if you have a tendency to develop urinary tract infections.

Method Two: Try using your fingers to feel the increase in tension when you contract your pelvic floor muscles. To do this:

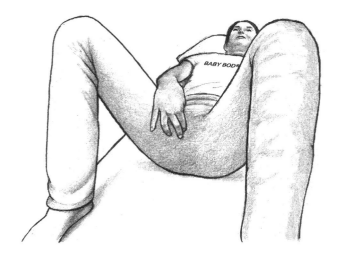

+ Lie on your back with your knees bent.

+ While wearing a pair of panties or thin workout pants, place your index and middle fingers on one side of the outside of the vagina (try the right side first). Make sure you are pressing into soft tissue. If it feels hard, you are pressing too far away from your vagina and into the pelvic bones, so move your fingers a little closer to your vagina and try it again. Use gentle pressure; do not press so hard that it causes pain. If you feel pain, STOP, and try it again with less pressure or wait a few days to try it again. (Please see the illustration above.)

- EXHALE gently and try doing a pelvic floor contraction by pretending you are stopping the flow of a *few drops of urine*.

- Hold it for 3 seconds and then relax. Can you feel the muscles tighten a bit under your fingers?

- Once you can feel a pelvic floor contraction on the right side, try feeling for a contraction on the left side.

- Make a mental note of how it felt to contract your pelvic floor, and how it felt once you relaxed it.

TIPS:

Tip 1: Imagine that you are trying to prevent passing gas. One of my favorite suggestions I tell my clients is to "Pretend you are in an elevator and your boss steps in and you feel like you are going to pass gas. What would you automatically do to prevent an embarrassing situation?" Yup, contract those pelvic floor muscles![A]

Tip 2: Don't be surprised if it feels as if one side is stronger than the other side; that's common and should even out with practice and time.

Tip 3: Don't worry if you can hardly feel a contraction during the first month or so after you delivered your baby. (The box below this section will help you understand why.)

Note: If you feel like you can hardly feel anything or just a little flicker, that's OK. Just continue to progress with the program. If you continue to feel unable to fully contract your pelvic floor muscles after you are about three months postpartum, it is time for you to seek treatment from a women's health physical therapist or physiotherapist.

[A] Lila Bartkowski Abbate PT, DPT, OCS, WCS, PRPC (www.new-dimensions-physical-therapy.com) came up with this visual, and it has helped tons of my clients understand how to contract their pelvic floor muscles. Thanks Lila!

Oh, no! I can't feel anything! Should I be worried?

Let me make something clear so you don't worry unnecessarily. *If you've recently given birth, don't be surprised if you don't feel much when you try to contract your pelvic floor muscles.* This is very common after birth because of the trauma your "lady parts" experienced from labor and delivery. In the beginning, you may feel a very slight contraction that seems to "flutter" and comes and goes. It's like having a lamp plugged into a faulty electrical socket, which flickers on and off. Don't worry! The strength of your contraction should improve with time if you follow the **Baby Bod® Program** in the correct sequence.

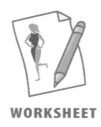

WORKSHEET

Try this little lesson before starting the Pelvic-Core Starter: Learn How to Prevent Creating a "Belly Bulge" When You Do the Pelvic-Core Starter

If you do the Pelvic-Core Starter exercise correctly, you should feel as if your lower tummy area is gently "scooping" or flattening, which may be a little difficult to feel at first, especially a month or two after childbirth. *I am not recommending that you "PULL" your belly button towards your spine!* The belly will flatten naturally, without effort on your part. When the core muscles are working optimally, they will automatically cause a natural "scooping" effect in the tummy. Don't try to force it by pulling your belly inwards! This will encourage the outer abdominal muscles to take over the work of the deeper core muscles and will work against your recovery.

To make sure you know what it feels like when your belly is bulging, I would like you to try the following *Belly Bulge Awareness Lesson*. This is what you should NOT feel when you do the Pelvic-Core Starter:

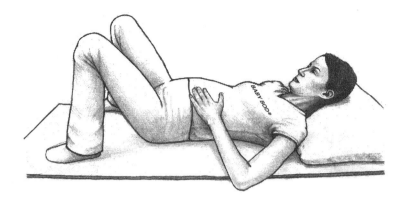

1. Lie on your back on a mat or mattress. (Yes, it's okay to do this if you are pregnant—you won't be on your back all that long.)

2. Place your hands on your lower tummy and lift your head and shoulders up off the mat.

3. You should feel your tummy bulging outwards. Let me repeat—this is NOT what you want when you do the Pelvic-Core Starter exercise.

Belly Flattening or Scooping – What you *should* feel when you do the Pelvic-Core Starter **exercise the correct way:**

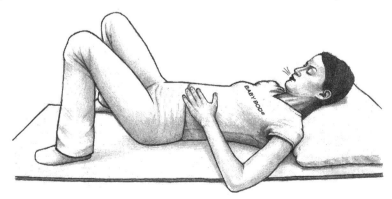

1. Place your hands on your lower tummy and lift your head and shoulders up off the mat. *(continues next page)*

2. Stay in the same position but before you lift up, align your chest with your pelvis, by making sure your rib cage it not tilted up towards the ceiling. Then EXHALE gently as you do a pelvic floor contraction and continue as you lift your head and shoulders up off the mat.

3. If things are working optimally, you should not feel your belly bulge and feel as if your lower tummy is scooping.

Remember this little exercise as you perform the Pelvic-Core Starter exercise.

The Safest Time to Start

When is it safe to start doing these? Most moms can start doing the Pelvic-Core Starter exercise the day after they deliver their baby, even if they had a C-section. Women who have had deep tears (Grade 3 or 4 tears)[B] in their vagina or pelvic floor area, however, need to wait until after the six-week checkup before starting. If you had any tears, it is best to first find out the degree of tearing that occurred and how much repair (stitching) was needed after delivery. Make sure to discuss this with your doctor or midwife and ask them if they think it is OK for you to start doing pelvic floor contractions now, or if they recommend waiting until the scar tissue heals, something that usually takes about six weeks.

> **Pelvic-Core Starter Exercises Can Help to Relieve Pain**
>
> Many of my clients have told me that doing the Pelvic-Core Starter exercise helps to relieve some of the initial cramping and discomfort that is common during the first few days after delivery. Performing these exercises helps to increase blood flow to the pelvic floor muscles, and this speeds healing.

[B] See "Perineal and Vaginal Tears" in Chapter 8 for more information about how tears in the pelvic region are graded.

When you do start performing the Pelvic-Core Starter, make sure not to cause pain. *If you are not pregnant* and find that any of these exercises are painful, STOP and wait a day or two before trying them again. Then try doing the exercise with less force. Only continue performing them if they don't cause pain.

If you are pregnant and experience pain while doing the Pelvic-Core Starter, STOP doing the exercises and report this to your doctor or midwife immediately. Only continue doing these exercises after you have medical clearance from your healthcare provider.

Pelvic-Core Starter: When Can I Start?	
If you're pregnant:	*Do the Pelvic-Core Starter pelvic-core starter any time throughout your pregnancy—until you're ready to give birth*—as long as it does not cause pain. Do NOT do these if your healthcare provider has cautioned you against doing any exercise. If you are permitted to exercise, DON'T do this exercise while lying on your back. Use the side-lying position instead.
If you had a vaginal delivery:	*Start the day after delivery*. (If you had a Grade 3 or 4 tear, follow the directions below.)
If you had a 3rd or 4th degree tear:	*Wait until after your six-week postpartum checkup* before starting the Pelvic-Core Starter exercises. If you get permission from your healthcare provider first, you can do most of the other **Preliminary Phase Exercises** during those first six weeks. But wait you are six weeks postpartum, before doing the **Straight Leg Raise Test** and the **Jumping Test**.
If you've had a C-Section:	*Start the day after surgery*, *unless you find it painful*. Do these gently enough so that they don't cause pain. If they do, stop and wait a day or two to resume. It's best to discuss this program with your doctor or surgeon before starting any of the exercises during the first six weeks after your surgery.
If it's been months or years since you've had your baby:	*Do the Pelvic-Core Starter and the other exercises in the Preliminary Phase for one week* before progressing to the more advanced exercises in the **Baby Bod® Program**.

THE PELVIC-CORE STARTER

Pelvic-Core Starter – Supine Position (Lying on Your Back):

You are going to first learn how to do this exercise while lying on a mat or even a mattress. After you understand how to do them correctly, I would like you to try doing them in different positions and then try to do them during simple daily activities, like when you are brushing your teeth, waiting for a pot of water to boil, or taking a walk.

Note: *If you are pregnant*, please use the side-lying position as you follow the directions below. Do not lie on your back.

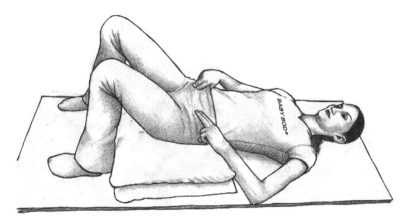

+ Lie comfortably on your back on a firm surface. Keep your head relaxed. Initially, you may use a pillow or two under your pelvis, if you like, so your buttocks are higher than your chest.

+ Bend your knees and hips, keeping your feet flat on the ground, hip-width apart.

+ Do your **Baby Bod® Alignment Check** and continue to stay in good alignment while you exercise. (If you need a good review, go back to Chapter Eleven.)

+ Place two fingers of each hand on the top part of your panty line, with your index and middle fingers gently resting on your panty line, just inside your pelvic bones.

+ Now, gently EXHALE and perform a pelvic floor contraction, as if you are trying to stop the flow of one or two drops of urine. (Not a bucket full!)

+ Try to hold this contraction for 3 seconds while slowly <u>counting out loud</u>, *"O-n-e Mississippi, T-w-o Mississippi, T-h-r-e-e Mississippi."*

+ Then relax the tension in your pelvic floor.

+ Then perform 3 quick contractions, where you gently contract then relax your pelvic floor, and <u>count out loud</u> with each contraction. (Try counting out loud by saying, *"One – Relax,"* *"Two – Relax,"* *"Three – Relax."*) Make sure to feel your pelvic floor relax a bit in between each quick flick.

+ Now relax for 6 seconds. Got It?

Week One:

Repeat this entire set (1 slow contraction and 3 quick flicks) 10 times, and rest for 6-seconds in between each set.

Do each set 10 times in a row, 3 times a day for one week and then progress as described below.

Week Two:

Progress to 4-second holds followed by 4 quick flicks and an 8-second rest.

Do each set 10 times in a row, 3 times a day for one week then progress as described below.

Week Three:

Progress to 5-second holds followed by 5 quick flicks and a 10-second rest.

Do each set 10 times in a row, 3 times a day for the remainder of this program.

Pelvic-Core Starter – Side-Lying Position:

If you are *pregnant or if find that it is difficult to perform the Pelvic-Core Starter while lying on your back,* try it lying on your side. Use a few pillows or a wedge to elevate your pelvis (see illustration below). Make sure to relax your tummy muscles and use your hand to feel your muscles relax in your lower tummy, and then slightly tighten when you contract your pelvic floor (then follow the directions above).

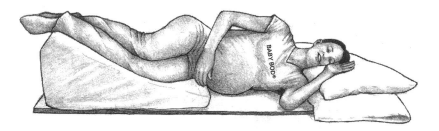

Try the Pelvic-Core Starter in Different Positions

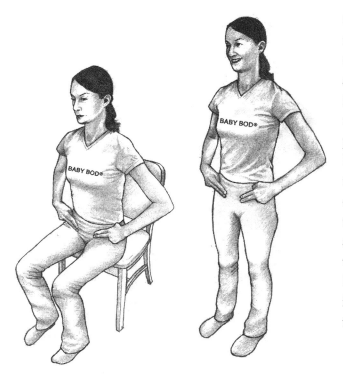

Once you feel confident about doing these exercises correctly, try doing them in different positions while *sitting, standing* and even *walking*. (Again, refer to the directions above; they're the same no matter what position you use.) Make sure to do the **Baby Bod® Alignment Check** prior to starting the Pelvic-Core Starter exercise in different positions. Then try to fit them in during normal daily activities, say, when you cook a meal, wait at a traffic light, or check your Facebook page. This way, you can fit in three full sessions three different times during the day.

Are You a Late Starter?

If it's been months or years since you've given birth, no worries: this program can work just as well for you. To get started, do the Pelvic-Core Starter and the other exercises in the Preliminary Phase for one week before progressing to the more advanced exercises in the Baby Bod® Program. You'll still derive a lot of benefit from them. They'll give your body the firm foundation it needs so it can once again be strong, healthy, and sexy.

And don't feel badly about starting so late. **"Once postpartum, always postpartum,"®** I say. This is a good way to prevent the kind of incontinence or pelvic pain that may have its roots in body changes during pregnancy or childbirth but takes a good five, ten, twenty years or more to fully manifest. [2]

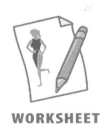

WORKSHEET

Cough Test [c]:

I would like you to stand and cough. What did you feel going on in your bottom? Try it again if you are not sure. Did you feel as if your pelvic floor dropped downwards? OK, that is normal. (*Record your results on your worksheet.*)

Now I would like you to contract your pelvic floor muscles by doing the Pelvic-Core Starter and holding it. Now COUGH. Did you feel your pelvic floor drop less? Good.

The point of this is to make you aware of how much more support you can offer your body when you actively do a pelvic floor muscle contraction. Try to remember to *contract* your pelvic floor prior to coughing, sneezing and laughing. And when exerting yourself, like picking up a laundry basket, heavy bag or even when you get up from a chair.

Majivecka/Shutterstock.com

---

[c] Special thanks to Sue Croft who gave me the idea to include the cough test in this book. She is a leader in women's health physiotherapy and practices in Queensland, Australia. (www.suecroftphysiotherapist.com.au)

Nine Tips for Success:

Tip 1: Make sure to feel as if your abdomen is gently drawing in towards your spine, not bulging outwards as you contract your pelvic floor muscles. (But don't "suck in" your gut!)

Tip 2: Don't hold your breath when you do the Pelvic-Core Starter. Instead, *count out loud* as you exercise. This will help you to exhale as you contract your pelvic floor muscles.

Tip 3: Don't forget to maintain the Baby Bod® Alignment Check position during the entire time you are doing the Pelvic-Core Starter exercise.

Tip 4: Remember to be gentle! Less is more. Your initial goal is to "wake up" the gentle holding fibers of the core muscles. If you get over zealous and try to squeeze with all your might, you will be working against yourself because you will be training the outer muscles and not the deep holders. [3]

Tip 5: Also make sure you stick to the *amount* of exercise I suggest. Don't assume that more is better and will get you faster results. It won't. Realize that pelvic floor muscles can become fatigued, just like any other muscle, and the progression of the exercises in **Baby Bod®** are based on scientific studies. [2] If you follow my directions, you are sure to get the best results possible.

Tip 6: Follow the timing I recommend. You will be training two different types of muscle fibers, ones that contract slowly and ones that contract quickly.

Tip 7: The Pelvic-Core Starter exercise should *feel* good. If you feel discomfort, try to do them more gently. You may find that your discomfort decreases after you've done the exercise two or three times. If, however, the pain continues or you feel an increase in pain or soreness, stop and wait a day or two before trying them again. (Please refer to Chapter Seven for some tips on how to relieve pelvic pain or muscle spasms.)

Tip 8: Are you having difficulty progressing with the Pelvic-Core Starter exercises? Try slowing down the progression, so that you progress every TWO weeks. By that, I mean continue to hold the slow contractions for three seconds followed by three quick flicks for TWO weeks, then progress to the four-second hold during weeks THREE and FOUR and five-second hold during weeks FIVE and SIX. If you still feel you are having difficulty progressing, you may have some muscles spasms or tightening in the pelvic floor muscles. Try out a few of the tips that are included in Chapter Seven on how to relieve muscle spasms and how to decrease pelvic pain. (Remember, don't be afraid to seek help by going to a women's health physical therapist or physiotherapist for a few visits.)

Tip 9: Ideally, the Pelvic-Core Starter exercises should be done on a daily basis. It is best to fit them in while you are performing other activities. But if you miss a day or two, don't sweat it. With busy moms, that's BOUND to happen. Just go back to it.

YAY! You did it! You just learned the BEST EXERCISE POSSIBLE to wake up your core muscles, speed your way to a flat tummy, and make sex more yummy! That's *if* you PRACTICE THEM DAILY!

Again, try to do three sets of the Pelvic-Core Starter exercises three different times a day.

How to Make the Most of the Pelvic-Core Starter

1. "Squeeze before your sneeze." To prevent urine leakage, try doing a *quick contraction* before you laugh, or when you feel a cough or sneeze coming on.

2. Try doing a quick contraction just before getting up from a chair or when you lift something heavy.

3. Try doing a series of Pelvic-Core Starter exercises to relieve back and pelvic pain.

* * *

Congratulations! You have now learned each of the **Preliminary Phase Exercises**. Where you are on the pregnancy to birth continuum will determine when you can start doing these daily and how long you need to continue this phase before you graduate to the **Advanced Phase–Strengthening Exercises**. As you know, I've covered that information in earlier chapters, but thought it would make things easier for you to include it here as well.

Determining Your Start and End Dates			
	When do I start?	**How long do I continue doing the Preliminary Phase Exercises before adding the Advanced Phase-Strengthening Exercises?**	**What precautions should I take?**
Pregnant	Today!	Up until you give birth	Avoid exercises that have you lie on your back.
Postpartum less than six weeks after giving birth vaginally, with no complications	24-48 hours after giving birth	Until after your 6-week checkup—as long as you get the "All OK" signal. Make sure to do at least one week of the Preliminary Phase Exercises prior to starting the Advanced Phase-Strengthening Exercises.	
Postpartum less than six weeks; had an episiotomy or have Grade 3 or 4 Tears	24-48 hours after giving birth	Until after your 6-week checkup—as long as you get the "All OK" signal. Make sure to do at least one week of the Preliminary Phase Exercises prior to starting the Advanced Phase-Strengthening Exercises.	Don't do the Pelvic-Core Starter until after you have your 6-week checkup, and get the "All OK" signal.
Postpartum less than six weeks after having a C-section	Please refer to the chart "Modified Preliminary Phase Exercises – C-section Moms" on page 172.	Until after your 6-week checkup—as long as you get the "All OK" signal. Make sure to do at least one week of the Preliminary Phase Exercises prior to starting the Advanced Phase-Strengthening Exercises.	Please refer to the chart "Modified Preliminary Phase Exercises – C-section Moms" on page 172.
Experienced moms well-past the 6-week postpartum checkup	Today!	Make sure to do at least one week of the Preliminary Phase Exercises prior to starting the Advanced Phase-Strengthening Exercises.	

Finally, don't forget that you can do the **Preliminary Phase Exercises** in bits and pieces throughout the day. My clients said they found this the easiest way to get everything done.

* * *

This completes the **Baby Bod® Preliminary Phase Exercises.** Please refer to Appendix B for a summary of the entire preliminary phase in chart form. Stick with this phase for the optimal amount of time that I mentioned in the chart above. When you're ready, turn the page and learn the **Advanced Phase—Strengthening Exercises** that you'll add to these exercises several days a week.

[1] Bump R, Hurt WG, Fantl JA, et al. Assessment of Kegel exercise performance after brief verbal instruction. *American Journal of Obstetrics and Gynecology.* 1991;165:322–329.

[2] Sapsford R. Rehabilitation of pelvic floor muscles utilizing trunk stabilization. *Manual Therapy.* 2004 Feb; 9(1):3-12.

[3] Hodges PW, Sapsford R, Pengel LH. Postural and Respiratory Functions of the Pelvic Floor Muscles. *Neurology and Urodyamics.* 2007; 26(3):362-371. doi: 10.1002/nau.20232.

Advanced Baby Bod® Exercises

If you've completed the **Baby Bod® Preliminary Phase** exercise program, your re-activated muscles are ready for a more challenging workout. In this chapter, I will teach you the **Advanced Phase—Strengthening Exercises**, which you will do for the next six weeks. If you do them conscientiously—three times a week—you'll love how your belly looks by the time you finish the program. You will be a lot stronger, too—inside and out!

Before I get to the specifics, here are few reminders. First, please remember to stay well hydrated, especially if you are breastfeeding your baby. Second, when you do these exercises, please pay special attention to the instructions on breathing and counting out loud. Follow them **exactly**. Remember that your core muscles work best when they work in coordination with each other; proper breathing helps synchronize the activity of all the muscles in your abdomen, which is what develops that flat tummy. The best way to make sure you are breathing correctly is to count out loud, which I will ask you to do. Counting out loud will ensure that your diaphragm muscle works in coordination with the rest of your core muscles.

Third, I want you to pay attention to your alignment. So if you jumped ahead and skipped Chapter Eleven on alignment, go back and make sure you know how to do the Baby Bod® Alignment Check, because it is the start position for all of these exercises.

Baby Bod® Alignment Check is the start position for all of these exercises.

Remember to stay well hydrated, especially if you are breastfeeding your baby.

Here's a brief summary of the **Baby Bod® Alignment Check** progression:

✓ Neutral pelvis position

✓ Straighten up from spine

✓ Exhale and stack chest over pelvis

✓ Shoulder roll

✓ Chin tuck

YOUR NEW ROUTINE

A lot of this will be familiar to you. I'd like you to continue doing the **Preliminary Phase Exercises** daily as before. In this advanced phase of the program, we're going to tweak them a bit. Now that you've moved to the advanced phase, this is what I want you to do:

1. **Baby Bod® Alignment Check.** Do daily. Use it to check your alignment (ideally) once an hour.

2. **Breathing Exercises.** Aim for once a day and do each exercise for 2 to 3 minutes. Alternate positions: Lying on back, sitting and standing.

3. **Warm Ups.** Do these daily.

4. **Walking Program.** Try to build up to daily 30-minute walks. Make sure to fit in two or three 10-minute walks on the days you are not able to do this.

"Kick starter" exercises encourage your core muscles to "kick in," or "wake up," so they work optimally.

5. **Pelvic-Core Starter Exercises.** First start with a 4-second hold, followed by 4 quick contractions and an 8-second rest in between each series. Then gradually progress to holding for 5 seconds, then 5 quick contractions and a 10-second rest. Do a total of 10 times, **three** times per day. Alternate positions: Lying on back, sitting and standing. (Note: It may take a few weeks to progress to holding for 5 seconds and 5 quick contractions.)

   If you are just starting to add the **Pelvic-Core Starter** to your recovery program because you had a *Grade 3 or 4 tear*, start with 3-second holds and 3 quick contractions and progress to 5-second holds over at least a 2-week period. Refer to Chapter Fourteen for full directions.

6. The **Advanced Strengthening Baby Bod® Exercises**, which I will teach you below. Do these 3 to 4 times a week.

THE FULL STRENGTHENING PROGRAM

We're going to start this program with two "kick starter" exercises, the Bow and the Stork. I call them "kick starters" because they help to "kick start" the muscles you will be targeting. In other words, they teach you how to use your body to encourage your core muscles to "kick in" or "wake up" so they work optimally. On the three days a week you do the full strengthening program, practice these first—a few times each—as a warm up before you do the strengthening exercises.

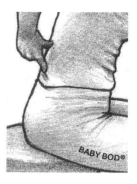

The Bow

This kick starter is important to learn for two reasons; first, it will help you use good form and keep good alignment when you exercise. Second, the Bow will teach you to bend at the hips and stop bending in the back. You need to be able to do this when you exercise and also during certain everyday activities, like when you bend down to get your baby out of the crib or groceries out of a shopping cart. Right now, I want to introduce the movement. In the next chapter, I will help you incorporate this smarter way of using your body into your everyday activities.

Practice this first while sitting in a chair, and then progress to doing the Bow in the standing position as a warm up to the strengthening exercises.

The Bow – Sitting Position

To start: Sit and get into good alignment by doing the Baby Bod® Alignment Check. Make sure that your chest is stacked over your pelvis. Then place your index finger and thumb on your lower back (see illustration above) and keep it there while you learn this movement. Use your fingers to monitor unwanted bending in your lower back.

- Stay in good alignment and then SLOWLY move your chest forward and towards your knees without rounding out your back. *Stop* if you feel your index finger and thumb spreading apart from each other and or you notice bending in your

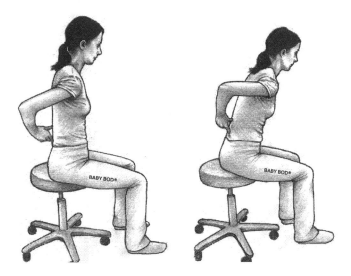

back. Then try it again. Move as if you are bowing forward.[A]

+ Try this several times in the seated position until you feel like you can bow without bending from your back.

+ First try it with your fingers monitoring the movement in your back. Then try it without using your fingers on your back.

Once you feel like you can do the Bow in sitting, try this while standing.

The Bow – Standing Position:

To Start: Stand and do a **Baby Bod® Alignment Check**, then place your index finger and thumb on your lower back and keep it there while you learn this movement. First practice the Bow standing with your fingers monitoring unwanted movement in your back and then progress to not using your fingers to monitor the motion, as in the illustration next page:

[A] It may be easier to do the Bow if you pretend that there is a stick on your back that extends from pelvis up to your skull. Try to bend without losing contact with the stick.

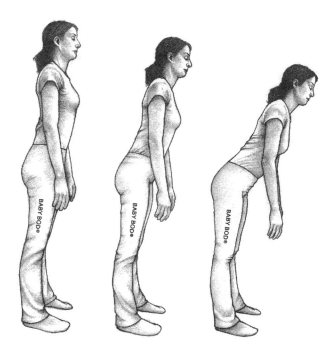

- Keep your knees slightly relaxed. Practice this once with your fingers on your back; in subsequent practice of this exercise, let your arms hang loosely.

- SLOWLY bend your torso forward, as if taking a bow, by bending only at the hips and not the back.

- Remember to drop your chest only about 8 to 12 inches and stop when you feel like you need to bend in the back. That's the normal amount. If you find that you can "fold over," you are probably bending at your back and doing the exercise wrong. More is not better here.

- Do **5** of these as a warm up before each of the strengthening exercise sessions.

The Stork

To Start: Stand with your side facing a chair and do a **Baby Bod® Alignment Check**. Place one hand on the chair for support. (If you don't have a stable chair handy, you can use a dresser or kitchen counter instead.)

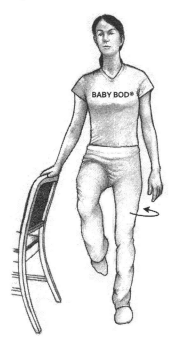

+ Lift the leg closest to the chair and keep your hip and knee bent.

+ Keep your body in the same position as you rotate your thigh away from the chair and hold it in this position for 10 seconds. *Count out loud* for 10 counts: *one Mississippi, two Mississippi*, etc. as you hold your thigh in the rotated position. (Make sure not to rotate your chest or pelvis. You should feel your buttock tighten on the side you are standing on as you hold your thigh in the rotated position.)

+ Do this **3** times on each leg as a warm up before each of the strengthening exercise sessions.

STRENGTHENING EXERCISES

Now let's move onto exercises specifically meant to strengthen your core and flatten your tummy. We'll begin with the Butt Lifter.

Butt Lifter

Strengthening exercises will strengthen your core and flatten your tummy.

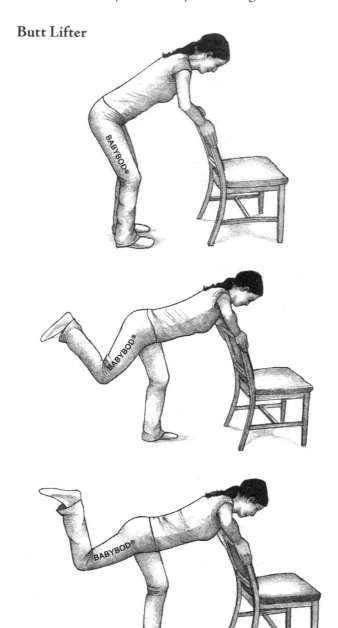

To Start: Stand facing the back of a chair and do a **Baby Bod® Alignment Check. Place your hands on the sides of the back of a chair.** (Make sure to place your hands down low enough so the chair does not tilt backwards.) Bend forward at the hips. Support some of your weight with your arms and maintain the Alignment Check position.

+ Bend one knee to 90 degrees and exhale as you lift your thigh up towards the ceiling and hold it in this position for 5 counts.[B] (**Count out loud** as you hold: *one Mississippi, two Mississippi,* etc. Make sure you don't rotate your pelvis or arch your back as you lift your leg).

+ Then keep your leg elevated and move your leg about 1 inch (3cm) up and down 5 times (do 5 pulses). (Count out loud as you pulse your leg, "ONE-UP, TWO-UP, THREE UP, etc.")

+ Return to start position and repeat 5 times with each leg.

The Bridge

To start: Lie on a mat with a thin pillow (or folded towel) to support your head and do a Baby Bod® Alignment Check.

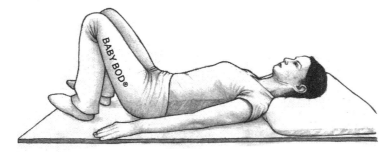

+ Bend your knees, hips and ankles. Press the heels of your feet into the mat and lift the balls of your feet off the mat with your toes pointing towards the ceiling.

[B] You will have the tendency to arch your back when you lift your leg. Maintain your **Baby Bod®** alignment by concentrating on using your butt muscle to lift your leg.

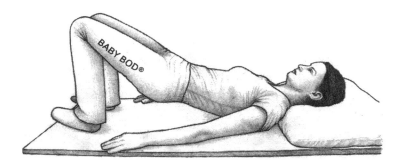

+ Exhale as you slowly lift your buttocks up off the mat, aiming for a straight line from your shoulders to your knees; make sure to keep your pelvis level and ribcage in line with your pelvis. Don't arch your back.

+ **Count out loud** as you hold this position for 5 seconds (5 *Mississippi's*).

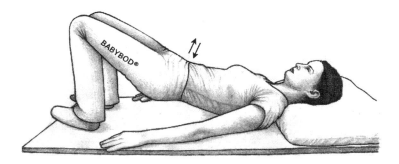

+ Remain in the bridge position and do 5 quick, short lifts as if you are moving or pulsing the pelvis up towards the ceiling 1 inch up and down 1 inch (3cm). **Count out loud** as you pulse your pelvis: "ONE-UP, TWO-UP, THREE-UP, etc."

+ Then slowly lower your body to the start position.

+ Do this series **5** times.

Heel Tapping and Heel Slides

The goal of this exercise is to be able to move your foot without rocking your pelvis. I am going to have you do it in two stages. Start by doing the *Heel Tapping* for at least a week, then progress to the next stage, *Heel Slides*. If you do find that your pelvis is moving when you try to progress, go back to doing Heel Tapping and continue for another week.

Heel Tapping

To Start: Lie on a mat with a thin pillow (or folded towel) to support your head.

Heel tapping can take a few weeks to master, so don't rush it. Good form is key here.

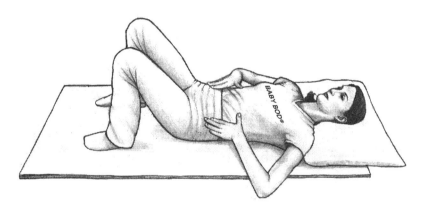

+ Bend your hips and knees and place your feet flat on the mat.

+ Do a **Baby Bod® Alignment Check.**

+ Then place your thumbs on the bottom of your rib cage and your fingers on the sides of the bony part of your pelvis. (Refer to the illustration above.) Keep your hands in this position throughout this entire exercise to monitor unwanted movement.

+ Gently exhale and lift one heel about 2 inches (5cm) off the mat and make sure not to wiggle your pelvis. Then keep your

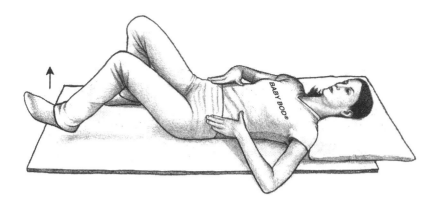

foot *above* the mat and move the foot a few inches away from your buttocks.

+ Start counting out loud (UP-One-Mississippi, DOWN-One-Mississippi, etc.) as you bring your knee towards your chest, and then return to the start position. Continue to monitor for unwanted movement and use your fingers to feel for this movement. If you find that you are rocking or wiggling your pelvis, STOP, and start over again. Try to decrease the amount you lift your leg. You may need to start this exercise by only moving your leg a few inches up and down and then progress to lifting more only when you can do this without moving or wiggling your pelvis.

+ Do this 10 times with each leg, one at a time. (Don't forget to *count out loud* each time you move your leg: "UP-One-Mississippi, Down-One-Mississippi, Up-Two-Mississippi, Down-Two-Mississippi, Up-Three-Mississippi, Down-Three-Mississippi," etc. until you finish doing it 10 times with each leg. Don't hold your breath.)

Heel Slides

Progress to doing Heel Slides after you have mastered the Heel Tapping and can do 10 taps with each leg without wiggling your

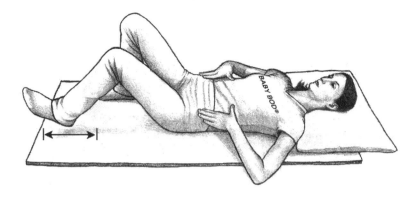

pelvis. It can take a few weeks, so don't rush it. Good form is key here.

- Start like you did with the Heel Tapping on a mat with both knees bent. Lift one of your heels 2 inches (5cm) above the mat and about 15-20 inches (40-50cm) away from your buttocks. Use your hands to monitor unwanted movement. Don't forget to exhale as you lift your foot.

- Count out loud, and instead of tapping, *keep your foot 2 inches (5cm) above the mat and try to slide it away from your body 5 to 10 inches (15-25cm)*. Then slide your foot back to the start position without touching the mat. (Make sure not to move your belly, pelvis or rib cage. Use your hands to feel for unwanted movement and don't forget to continue to count in Mississippis the entire time you do this exercise.)

- Continue moving back and forth without touching 10 times. (If you feel your pelvis rocking, stop and restart again. Try to decrease the amount you "slide" your foot above the mat. You may need to start this exercise by only moving your foot an inch or two (2.5 to 5 cm) and then progress to "sliding" it longer distances only when you can do this without moving your pelvis.)

Side-Leg Glides

To Start: Learn this well, because you will be using this as the start position for several of the mat exercises below.

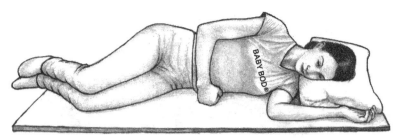

+ Lie on your side with a folded pillow or towel roll under your head for support.

+ Do a **Baby Bod® Alignment Check.** Make sure to have your head supported so that your spine is straight. (Imagine looking at your body from the back and seeing your entire spine straight, like in one of those memory foam mattress commercials.)

+ Place your upper arm against your tummy as if you are hugging yourself, and then stiffen your wrist and make a fist. Gently press your fist into the mat, making sure to keep your wrist straight. Continue pressing into the mat during the entire exercise.

+ Keep the upper arm in this position and gently pull your shoulder blade towards the middle of your back where you have your bra clasp. Stay in this position while doing this exercise.

+ Bend both of your legs so the hip is at a 45-degree angle and the knees at a 90-degree angle. (Refer to the illustration above.)

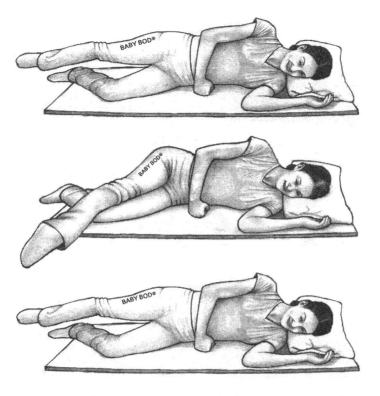

+ Then straighten your top leg and lift it to hip height (NOT higher).

+ Then exhale and count out loud (in Mississippis) as you move the top leg forward while keeping the knee straight. Stop when you feel tension in the back of your thigh.

+ Then move your straight leg back until it is lined up in a straight line with the rest of your body, the start position. Don't try to move your leg backwards, behind your body. Make sure to keep your knee straight throughout the entire glide.

+ Do this **15** times with each leg.

Note: It is OK to start out only doing a *smaller partial glide*. Move only until you feel tension in the back of your knee or thigh and stop at that point and return to the start position. This exercise targets the muscles in your buttock. If you try to move beyond your natural flexibility, you will be forcing yourself to use bad form and strengthen the wrong set of muscles. Don't get discouraged; in time and with practice you will get there. If you continue moving in easy ranges, your body will slowly gain more flexibility and you will eventually be able to glide in larger arcs of movement.

Also, as you do this, realize the importance of paying attention to how you hold your pelvis. *DON'T ROLL YOUR PELVIS BACKWARDS!* A lot of people have the tendency to do this when they move their legs backwards. You can use your arm to monitor this: If you feel your body move away from your arm, you are rolling your pelvis backward. If this happens, *stop*, and start the exercise again.

Leg Circles

To Start: Get into the same start position as the start position for the Side-Leg Glides. (page 284)

- Straighten your top leg and lift it to hip height (NOT higher).

- Exhale and count out loud as you move your straight leg in 10 little circles clockwise and then 10 counter-clockwise. (Imagine tracing your big toe in circles the size of a silver dollar.)

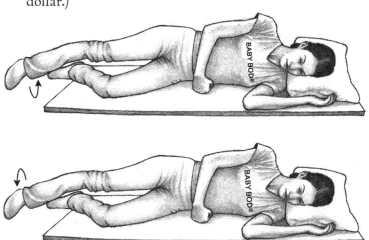

Underneath Side Leg Lifts

To Start: Get into the same start position as the start position for the Side-Leg Glides. (page 284)

+ Bend your top leg at the hip and knee so they are bent at 90-degree angles. Touch the mat with the bent knee.

+ Straighten your bottom leg, knee and hip and keep it straight the entire time you are doing this exercise.

+ Exhale and count out loud as you raise your leg up and down about one or two inches or 5cm (no more) 20 times with each leg. This is a faster lift, so do it as if you are pulsing up and down for a count of 1, 2, 3, 4, etc., not slowly.

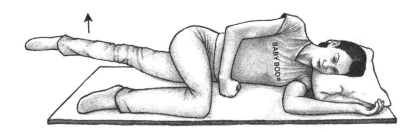

Knee Touch Downs

To Start: Get into the same start position as the start position for the Side-Leg Glides (page 284), with your hips bent at a 45-degree angle and the knees at a 90-degree angle. Then:

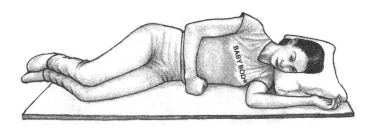

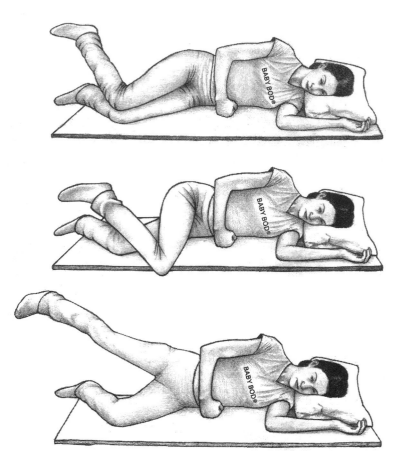

+ First, with your thighs touching, lift the foot of the upper leg towards the ceiling. (Do this by rotating your thigh towards your other thigh. It should feel as if you are turning your kneecap towards the inside.)

+ Keep your knee bent and bring it down and forward and touch the mat with your knee.

+ Then bring your leg back until your straight leg is lined up with your body and above hip height. (Make sure not to roll your pelvis backwards as you lift your leg.)

+ Exhale and count out loud as you move and do 10 times with each leg.

Table Top – Rib Expanders

To Start: Get on your hands and knees on the mat. Take your shoes and socks off for this exercise. Keep your ankles bent and toes flexed (curled under). Turn your hands so that your fingers are facing each other. Align your hips over your knees and your shoulders over your hands. Do a Baby Bod® Alignment Check and make sure your head, chest, and pelvis are in a straight line.

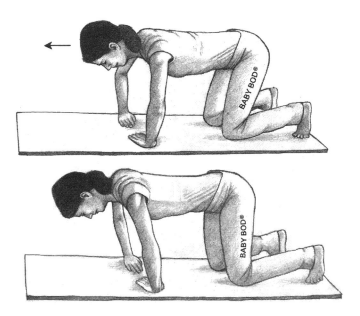

+ Bend your elbows slightly.

+ Keep your feet, knees, and hands planted on the mat as you move your body forward, so that your breasts and not your shoulders are over your hands. Try to keep your spine straight, with your head in line with your spine, the entire time you are doing this exercise.

+ Stay in this position and practice your rib expander breathing (without using an old tie) while you hold this forward position for 15 seconds. *(continues next page)*

♦ Repeat holding this position for 15 seconds 2 times. Gradually build up the amount of time you can hold this position until you can hold it for 30 seconds, 2 times in a row.

Notes: If you experience pain turning your hands towards each other, don't turn them as much. If this happens, you will need to do more of the Bali Dancer Nerve Glide exercises I taught you earlier to get yourself ready for turning your hands inwards.

Side Planks
To Start: Lie on your side with your hips and thighs straight and knees bent at a 90-degree angles. Do a **Baby Bod® Alignment Check** and prop yourself up on your elbow.

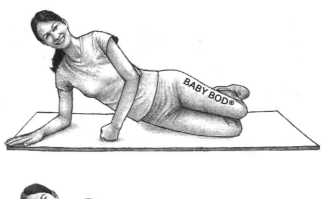

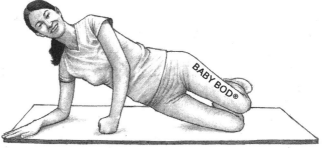

♦ Push your body up towards the celling by pressing down with your fist (see illustration). Keep your hips straight and don't rotate your torso.

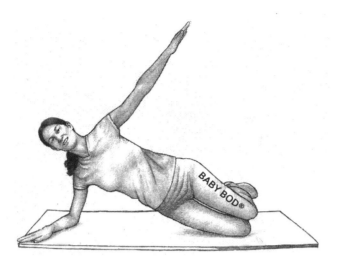

+ Keep your body in a straight line and lift your arm up towards the ceiling.

+ Hold this position for 15 seconds while counting out loud. Repeat 2 times on each side.

+ Gradually build up the amount of time you can hold this position until you can hold it for 30 seconds and repeat 2 times on each side.

Chair Squats

To Start: Place a stable chair against a wall for support; don't use a computer chair with wheels at the bottom. Make sure to wear sneakers or keep your feet bare with this exercise to prevent slipping when you squat. Stand facing away from the chair with your legs about 6 to 8 inches (17-23cm) away from the seat. Do a **Baby Bod® Alignment Check.** (*continues next page*)

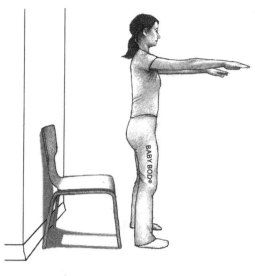

To Squat:

+ With your hands straight out in front of you, do the Bow.

+ Then continue to bend by pushing your buttocks backwards as you bend your hips and knees.

+ Slowly do a squat until you sit on the chair.

Note: *You may need to use a yoga block or large book to increase the height of the chair to make it easier when you are first learning how to do chair squats.*

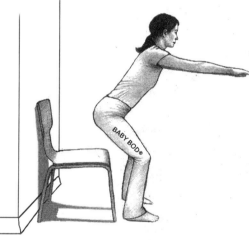

To Get Up:

+ Move to the edge of the chair with your feet flat on the floor.

+ Place your hands in front of you like Superman.

+ Do the Bow in the seated position; bend at your hips and not your lower back.

+ Press down on your forefoot as you rise out of the chair. Try getting up in the bow position, imagining how your body feels when you jump off a diving board. Do not bring your body straight up towards the ceiling. Once you are about three-quarters of the way up, you can straighten up your body.

+ Try to do 10 of these in a row.

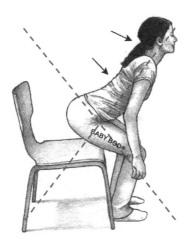

Chair Squats: How to Get Your Form Correct

When you are doing Chair Squats, make sure not to arch your neck or back. Keep your head aligned over your chest and chest over pelvis the entire time you do this exercise.

Standing Squats

Progress to doing a squat without using a chair. Continue to wear sneakers or perform the squats with bare feet. Remember to stay aligned and to exhale or count out loud as you squat down and as you straighten up.

Do 10 times.

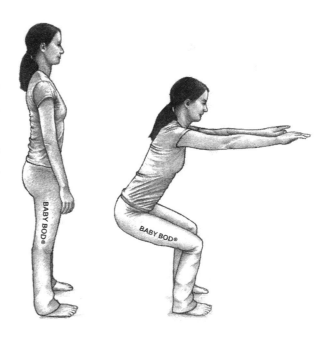

Salt-Water Taffy Pulls

Salt-Water Taffy Pulls - Sitting:
   To start: Sit on a hard chair with a stable base, not a chair with wheels or couch. Do a **Baby Bod® Alignment Check.**

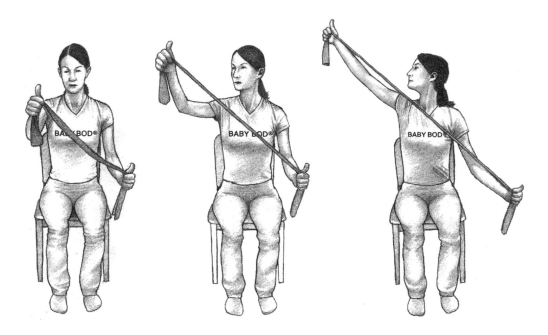

+ Grasp an exercise band and point your thumbs up, letting the ends dangle.

+ In the front of your body place one hand at shoulder level, and the other below your waist. Maintain constant eye contact with the thumb on your upper hand throughout this entire exercise.

+ Start counting out loud as you move both arms in opposite diagonal directions. Straighten both elbows as you raise and lower your arms.

+ Stop when arms are straight and the exercise band touches your chest.

+ Return to the start position.

+ Repeat this 15 times on each side.

Salt-Water Taffy Pulls – Standing

When you have been doing this program for **at least three weeks**, progress to doing the salt-water taffy pull while standing. (Repeat 15 times on each side.)

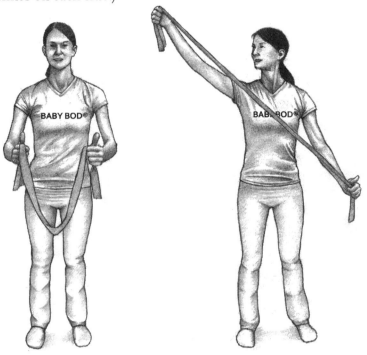

Note: You should be able to do this with just a little effort. If you find this hard to do, first practice it without using the exercise band, then start with a large "loop" of exercise band in between your hands. As you get stronger, you can shorten the size of the loop. This will increase resistance. Keep in mind, however, that it is better to do these exercises with good form and less resistance rather with more resistance and bad form.

Here's what I mean by **bad form**: Don't arch or lift your chest, or arch your neck when doing this exercise. If you find that you are doing this, lighten up the resistance.

Well, that's it for the **Advanced Phase—Strengthening Exercises**. Do these for six weeks to complete the **Baby Bod® Program**.

IF YOU WANT TO RETURN TO THE GYM . . .

If you belong to a gym and you miss it, now is a good time to go back, as long as you don't get too crazy. Do your **Baby Bod® exercises** on the mat. I recommend that you wait until you have finished this program before starting a more aggressive exercise program. If you have a trainer, ask them to follow this program and spot you while you progress with this program.

If you want to increase the amount of calories you are burning and get a good workout for your heart, add intervals of low-impact cardio exercises in between these exercises. Just avoid "jarring" moves; you shouldn't jump or run until you pass the Straight Leg Raise Stability Test and the Jumping Test (see these tests in Chapter Five).

Here's my take on other possibilities at the gym:

Stationary Weight Machines: I do not recommend these since they eliminate stabilization training. You'd be better off working to increase your strength by using free weights, exercise bands, and a cable column. Steer clear of heavier weights for now. Also avoid high resistance; it is better to use good form and work out with lower weights and use higher repetitions.

Treadmill: It's fine to walk on the treadmill when you first return to the gym and gradually build up the speed to fast walking. Start off by using a slight incline; you can gradually increase the incline as you build up your endurance. Please wait until you are at least three months postpartum and can pass the Straight Leg Raise Stability Test and the Jumping Test (see Chapter Five) to start running on one.

Stationary Bike: This is okay as long as it is not painful to sit on the bike seat. You may be more comfortable using a recumbent bike instead of an upright bike.

The Elliptical: For the first three months after you give birth, stick with low resistance and a smaller arch or incline. I also recommend that you hold the side rail instead of using the moving arms.

A Word of Caution to the Serious Athletes/Extreme Exercisers Among You

Yes, I know. You're chomping at the bit to do whatever you exceled in before you became pregnant. Just don't push it. An injury now could set your recovery back. That's why I advise you to wait until at least three months after you've had your baby AND until you can pass the Straight Leg Raise Test and Jumping Test (see Chapter Five) to return to activities, exercises or sports that involve high impact, running, jumping, and/or heavy lifting. If you find a Pelvic/SI Belt is helpful when you perform these tests, try using a belt when you exercise. Please refer back to Chapter Five for more information on this.

GROUP CLASSES

Group classes can provide you with a terrific way to spend some time with other adults, provided you use common sense and realize that your needs as a pregnant or postpartum woman might be different than those of the woman exercising next to you. Here's my advice.

Yoga classes: Don't overstretch or push the end ranges until you are at least three months postpartum. If you are nursing your baby, you need to use caution until three months after you wean your child.

Group Exercise: You can start lower-impact classes after your six-week checkup. Try to wait until you are three months postpartum before starting higher impact classes that require weights, running and jumping activities. If you are nursing your baby, you need to use caution until three months after you wean your child.

Spin Class: Try to wait until you are three months postpartum before starting spin classes. It is important to make sure that you DON'T hold your breath, which will increase the pressure in your belly and can stress the connective tissue connecting the rectus abdominis muscles and/or strain your pelvic floor muscles.

* * *

That's it for the exercise program, but it's not the end of **Baby Bod**®. How would you like to do your back and neck a big favor? In the next two chapters, I'll teach you body-smart ways to shop for—and use—routine baby gear, like your changing table, car seat carrier, and stroller.

CHAPTER SIXTEEN

Baby Gear That's Great for Your Body, Too[1]

Remember the children's story "Goldilocks and the Three Bears"? Shopping for baby gear like strollers, baby carriers and nursery furniture can be a little like that. One will be too big, another too small, and the third will be *just right*—for your baby, your budget, and YOUR body.

I put the emphasis on YOUR body because few moms (or their partners) give this much thought. Typically, when most people think of *ergonomics* they tend to think of office chairs or workplace design and how it affects their back, neck or wrists. It doesn't occur to most parents to think about the *ergonomic design of baby equipment, OR how the design or size* of the baby gear they use on a daily basis could have an adverse effect on their bodies.

Luckily for you, I've thought about this a LOT. Taking care of your child can cause a lot of stress and strain on your body. If you aren't moving correctly and using gear that supports your back, neck, shoulders, and/or joints, you could end up developing lots of aches and pains that are preventable. I would like to give you a few tips on how to prevent aches and pains by choosing the best baby gear for *your* body and how to use it correctly. In this chapter, I'm going to provide you with a set of guidelines you can use when you are considering buying or acquiring baby gear from a relative or friend.

Prevent aches and pains by choosing the best baby gear for your body and using it correctly.

If you've been conscientiously following the **Baby Bod® Program**, you have extra reason to consider your own body when you buy baby gear. You know that each time you correct your alignment you're helping the muscles that hold in your tummy work more efficiently, right? So why would you want to use gear that takes your body *out* of alignment?

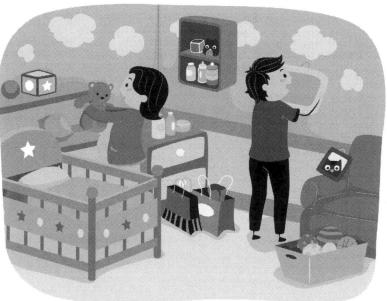

THE NURSERY [2]

Crib

Before 2011, crib manufacturers sold cribs with drop-down sides. These were easier on the back because you could drop the side down instead of having to bend over the crib to lift baby out. After those cribs were blamed for the deaths of thirty-two babies between 2000 and 2010, the U.S. Consumer Product Safety Commission banned the sales of cribs with drop-down sides.

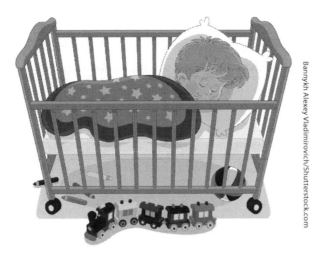

Bannykh Alexey Vladimirovich/Shutterstock.com

The cribs on the market now have stationary sides. Most cribs will let you change the height of the crib mattress by lowering the mattress support. This way, when your child gets bigger and begins sitting up, or begins to pull up or stand, you can lower the mattress so that your child can't climb or fall out of the crib.

That keeps your baby safe. The deeper the mattress, however, the more you have to bend and the greater the risk of straining your back. Fortunately, there's a simple way to protect your back. Keep a footstool near the crib. When you're ready to lift your baby from the crib, place one foot on the stool first. That will take the strain off your back. Or if you are petite, you might find it easier to stand on the stool as you reach in to lift your child.

Footstool

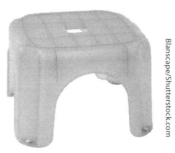

Blanscape/Shutterstock.com

One of the best pieces of advice I can give you is to buy a few inexpensive footstools about nine inches (23cm) tall and fifteen inches (38cm) wide to use in the nursery and other areas of your home. They have lots of uses. You can use one *near the changing table,* and you can also use it to sit on when you *sit down on the floor* to play with your toddler. If you choose to sit on the floor, you can place a hand on the step stool and push down on it as you get up from the floor. It's also a good idea to keep a step stool *near the kitchen sink* and *anywhere else you spend a lot of time bending over.* You always want to think about taking care of your back and using good alignment as you go through your daily activities.

Changing Table

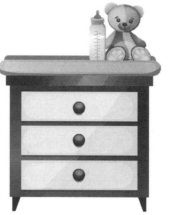

Ideally, the *height of the changing table* should be slightly below your elbows. If you can't find one at the right height for you, you can relieve stress on your back by placing a footstool near the table and placing one foot on the stool while changing your child. If you are tall, try adding a thick pad to raise the height of the table. Or if you are shorter, try standing on the stool.

Position the changing table in the room so that you can stand directly in front of it. This will help you avoid the type of bending and twisting that can strain your back.

Be sure to keep the *supplies* you need to change the diapers are in easy reach, such as on the top shelf or top drawer of the changing table. Another option is to put a shelf above the changing table. Position it so that it's easy to reach, but high enough to give you enough room to change the baby. For most people, this will be roughly 2-3 feet (60-90cm) above the table, but the exact measurement depends upon your height.

Comfortable Chair

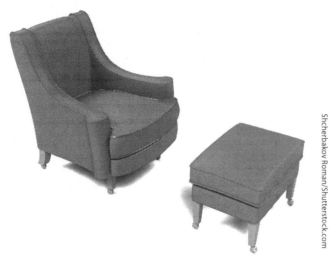

Shcherbakov Roman/Shutterstock.com

Another essential a mom can't do without is a comfortable chair you can sit in while nursing or feeding your baby. Since you'll spend many hours a day feeding your newborn, it is best to find a chair that offers lower back support and arm rests. A recliner might be a good choice because it also offers support for your legs and feet. Alternately, you can choose a chair that has a separate footstool or ottoman.

If you already have a chair, you may need to add additional pillows to support your back and arms. A *nursing pillow*, which you put on your lap, can be used to support your baby and prevent you from hunching over during feedings.

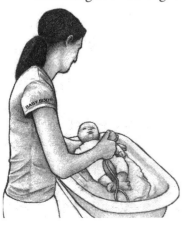

Baby Bath Tub

It's easier on your back to use a "baby bathtub" to bathe your child instead of bending down to bathe your baby in a standard-sized bathtub. Some are sized to fit right in your kichen or bathroom sink or on top of a counter. You can find baby bathtubs in many department stores and children's specialty shops.

CARRIERS AND STROLLERS
Front Baby Carriers

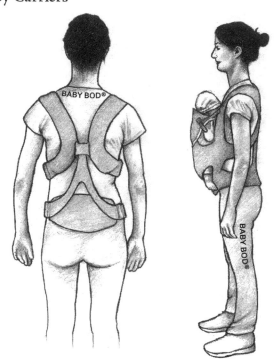

Front carriers can be great for your baby and you; they free up your hands so you can get things done. But make sure you get an adjustable one so that it fits you correctly. (If you can't adjust your baby carrier to fit your body, then it is the wrong style of baby carrier for you. Return it.) Be sure to follow the manufacturer's directions, especially the precautions about when it is safe to start using it. Certain carriers can be used when the infants are small and others aren't meant to be used until the child is a few months old.

I see moms and dads walking with front baby carriers almost every day in Manhattan… and most of them are using them incorrectly. Here's how to adjust your baby carrier so you can rest assured that you are supporting the baby's weight with your pelvis and legs, rather than your back:

The *bottom of the baby carrier* should go down low enough so that the belt wraps around the bony parts on the sides of your pelvis. If the belt is placed correctly, it will transfer the weight off

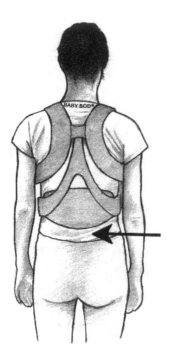

the shoulders and back and on to the hips and legs. The fit should be tight enough so that the carrier does not ride up. Make sure the *shoulder straps* fit over the middle of your shoulders. They should not be too close to your neck nor sliding down off your shoulders. What I often see is that the carrier belt is up too high and sitting above the pelvis, which places a strain on the back.

Question: Take a look at the illustration below. After reading the advice I just gave you, can you figure out what's WRONG with wearing the carrier like this?

Answer: This is fitted incorrectly because the length of the baby carrier is too short and the belt is not wrapped around the pelvis. Also, the straps are too close to the neck and could possibly cause some neck and shoulder pain. Make sure the front carrier you choose is long enough to have the belt wrap around your pelvis and not your waist. And again, as I said above, make sure the *shoulder straps* fit over the middle of your shoulders rather than sitting too close to your neck or sliding down off your shoulders.

Carry your baby so that the baby's head is below your chin. This height will give you enough room to move around comfortably and will help keep the weight of the baby close to your center of gravity.

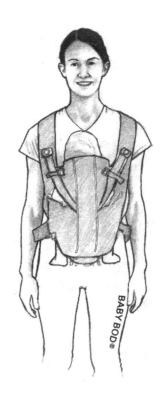

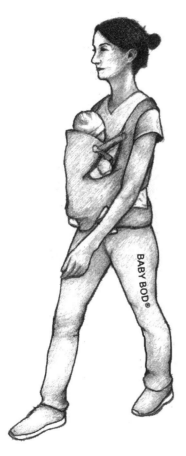

If you are wearing the baby carrier correctly, you should be able to walk while maintaining good alignment and with a normal, comfortable stride.

If you do use a front carrier, make sure to continue to use good alignment and do your **Baby Bod® Alignment Check** right after you place the baby into it. Try to do some Alignment Checks every so often to make sure you are moving, standing and walking in the best way possible to prevent straining your back and neck.

Each product has its own set of directions. Be sure to read them. (If you are going to a physical therapist for treatment, bring in your baby carrier and ask your therapist to fit it for you.)

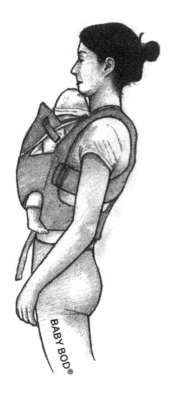

Question: Can you tell what's wrong in the illustration?

Answer: Mom is not aligned and is standing with poor posture. Also, the carrier is too high: the baby's head is up against the mom's chin, and the belt is too high and not wrapped around the pelvis.

Baby Stroller

If you're buying a new baby stroller, don't buy it based on looks but on how it fits your body. It should be the right size for your height and promote a comfortable stride. The height of the handle should allow your arms to be fairly straight and slightly bent at the elbows. If you are tall, look for a stroller that has an adjustable handle or one that has been designed to accommodate handle extenders. (There are also some "universal" handle extenders you can buy.) If you're short, look for a stroller that is smaller.

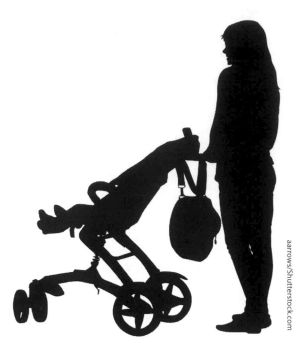

aarrows/Shutterstock.com

You'll know if your stroller fits if you can push it and you can:

- Keep your head and chin up, and your ears above your shoulders.

- Keep your shoulders down and back, leading with your chest and staying as close to the stroller as possible.

- Keep your arms slightly bent (don't lock them).

- Keep your wrists straight when you are holding the handlebars.

- Engage your whole body, not just your arms, through all movements.

No matter your height, make sure the stroller allows you to easily put your diaper bag on it so you don't have to carry it on your shoulder. There are stroller hooks and cup holders you can purchase if your stroller doesn't have this.

If you live in an urban area, do your research to find the best models for urban dwellers. There are numerous articles on this—with real reviews—on the web. You want one that can easily navigate curbs and those unexpected cracks in the sidewalks.

If your budget allows, there's a very expensive stroller that looks like an egg, with an adjustable seat that glides up and down. That's ideal because when the baby is little, you can adjust the seat up higher to make it easier to take your baby in and out of it. As your child gets older, bigger, and heavier, you can make the seat lower, which makes it easier for them to crawl into it and step out of it without you having to lift them up.

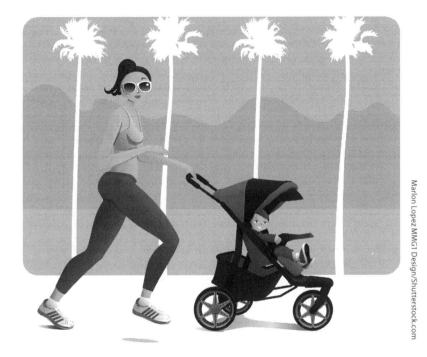

Marlon Lopez MMG1 Design/Shutterstock.com

If you plan to jog with the stroller, get a stroller specifically made for jogging. [3] Look for a lightweight jogging stroller, since lifting and carrying heavy objects can be hard on the lower back, especially if you do it incorrectly. In the next chapter, which focuses on how to move correctly, I'll explain how to run with the stroller so that you don't injure yourself.

* * *

Happy—and smart—shopping! In the next and final chapter, we'll look at how to get your **Baby Bod®** *On All Day Long*, as you take care of your baby throughout the day. Master these few moves, and that flat tummy—and pain-free back and neck—will be yours!

[1] APTA. Painless Parenting 101. Move Forward. http://www.moveforwardpt.com/resources/detail.aspx?cid=610b67e1-3d67-4ce9-a5b1-06c0c058fa66#.VHzyhkktDIU. Published April 25, 2013.

[2] APTA. Ergonomic Parenting: Best Ways to Prepare or Adapt to your Nursery. Move Forward. http://www.moveforwardpt.com/resources/detail.aspx?cid=3cb64c31-3803-4f97-b516-b87fa7e3d5db#.VHz1dEktDIU. Published May 7,2013.

[3] FIT4MOM. Safe Strides: Jogging Stroller Safety Tips. http://fit4mom.com/latest/blog/safe-strides-jogging-stroller-safety-tips.

Get Your Baby Bod® On All Day Long

Congratulations! You've learned almost everything I set out to teach you with my **Baby Bod® Program** and I bet you're well on your way to a stronger, sexier body. Just make sure you're still checking your alignment several times a day and remembering to exhale when you exert yourself! I also want you to go back and review the Bow exercise, which is in Chapter Fifteen. You'll need to know it to do some of the movements in this chapter correctly.

There's just one more little bit to teach you and yes, it's as critical as everything else you've learned in this book.

In Chapter Six, I explained how good alignment encourages your core muscles to automatically hold your tummy in and support your body. If most of your day involves caring for a new baby—or doing anything else for that matter—that will only take you so far. You also need to know how to *stay* in right alignment when you move, and by that I mean each time you lift the baby to feed, burp, and cuddle, or bend down to change and bathe the baby, etc.

Does this mean you can skip this chapter if you're an experienced mom who had her last baby years ago? Nope. I want you to read this chapter as well. What I explain below about how to properly lift something and hold a heavy object also applies to you. Learning to move correctly throughout the day—no matter where you are on the birth continuum—is the best way to flatten that "Mommy Tummy" and prevent the aches and pains that can arise when you're making the same moves again and again.

You need to know how to stay in right alignment when you move.

As I tell my clients, "You need to get your **Baby Bod**® on ALL DAY LONG." So let's look at how to do just that!

LIFTING

If you were to stop and count the number of times per day you lift your baby, you'd probably be surprised at how high the number is. Since this is a move you repeat often every single day, you definitely want to learn how to do this with the least amount of effort and in a way that prevents strain on your body.

Lifting Baby Out of a Crib

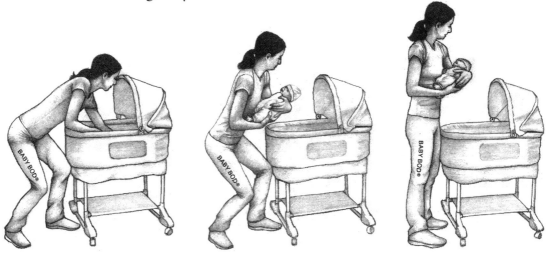

Here's the step-by-step for **picking up your child from a crib:**

1. Stand close to the crib and right next to where your child is resting to avoid twisting your back.

2. Keep your feet shoulder width apart and knees slightly bent. You can place one foot in front of the other foot, as in a mini-lunge position (refer to the illustration above). Or you can place one foot on top of a stool to prevent straining your lower back.

3. Make sure you are in good alignment by centering your rib cage over your pelvis prior to bending over. (If you need to, reread the **Baby Bod® Alignment Check** review in Chapter Eleven.)

4. Bend at your knees and hips, not your back. Do the Bow exercise (see Chapter Fifteen) and continue bending in the hips and knees until you feel you can get a secure grasp on your child.

5. EXHALE as you lift your child with both arms and bring the baby close to your chest.

6. Then straighten your knees and hips to return to a full standing position.

7. Keep your child close to your chest as you carry him or her around.

DON'T Do This:

Now that you've read the guidelines I've just given you, see if you can answer this question:

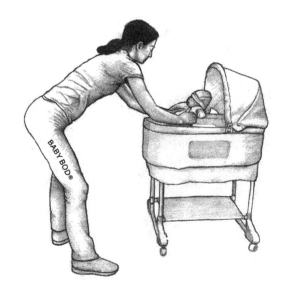

Question: What is wrong with the way the woman in the illustration is lifting the baby from the crib?

Answer: She is not close enough to the crib. She is bending too much in her back and not enough in her knees. This will increase strain on her lower back.

Lifting Baby Out of a Stroller

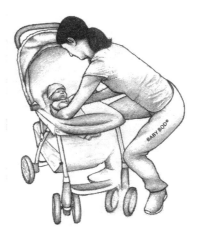

Picking your baby up out of a stroller is similar to picking your baby up out of a crib. Before you pick up your baby, however, make sure to lock the stroller wheels and get rid of any bags you are carrying. Then follow the directions above on how to lift.

DON'T Do This:

Question: What is wrong with the illustration below?

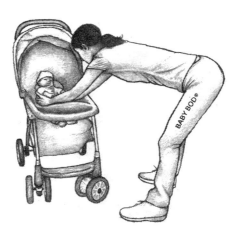

Answer: Mom is too far away from the stroller; she is bending too much in her back and her knees are not bent. She risks straining her back.

Lifting Baby Out of a Car Seat

You can also use this same lifting technique when you lift your baby out of a car seat. (Refer to the directions mentioned earlier.) Just make sure to bring your body close to the car seat before lifting.

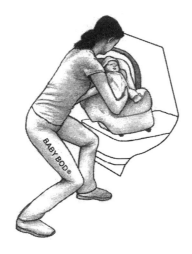

DON'T Do This:

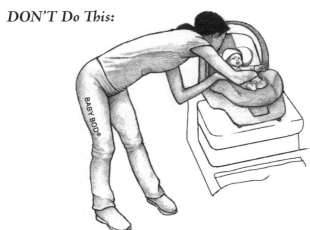

Question: Can you find three things wrong with the way the woman in the illustration below is lifting her baby out of a car seat?

Answer: She is standing too far away from the car seat, twisting her body, and bending her back, rather than her knees. She needs to stand in closer and bend from her knees rather than bending and twisting her back.

Lifting the Baby in a Baby Carrier

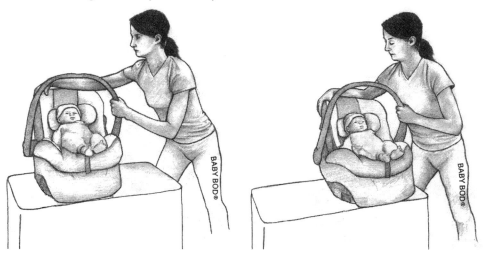

Try not to carry any other bags when you lift your baby in a baby carrier. Put them down first. When you lift your baby in a carrier:

- Stand directly in front of the seat to avoid twisting your back.

- Keep your feet shoulder width apart and knees slightly bent. You can place one foot in front of the other foot, like in a mini-lunge position.

- Make sure you are in good alignment by centering your rib cage over your pelvis prior to bending over.

- Bend at your knees and hips, not your back. Do the Bow and continue bending in the hips and knees until you feel you can get a secure grasp on the baby carrier.

- Slide the carrier closer to your body.

- Place your hands on either end of the seat, as if you were carrying a basket of laundry. Try not to lift the carrier from the center handle.

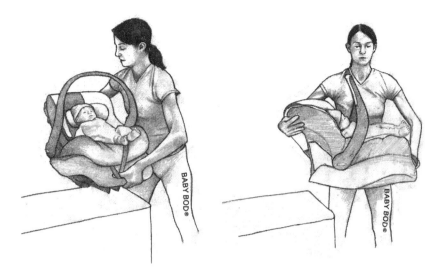

- ✦ Make sure you are in good alignment by centering your rib cage over your pelvis prior to bending over.

- ✦ EXHALE as you lift the baby carrier.

- ✦ If you need to turn, turn your entire body by circle stepping with your feet or pivoting with your feet; don't twist your back.

When you need to put down a car seat or baby carrier, try doing the reverse.

DON'T Do This:

Question: Can you find three things wrong in the illustration?

Answer: Mom is talking on the phone, not facing the carrier and using only one hand to pick the baby up.

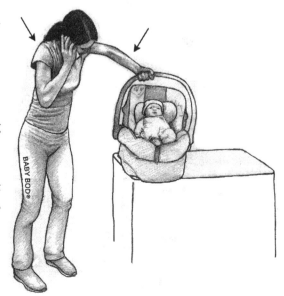

Lifting Your Baby or Something Else off the Floor

When you have a baby or toddler, you'll do a lot of bending down to pick up the baby, toys, laundry, etc. Doing it the right way can prevent aches and pains. Here are my best tips.

Golfer's Lift:

To pick up a toy or piece of laundry off the floor, try using the "Golfer's Lift" to avoid straining your back.

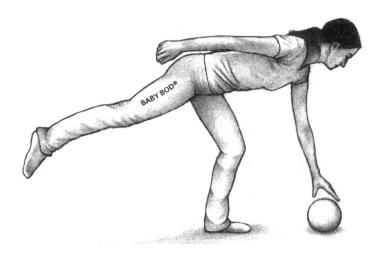

1. Stand close to the object and make sure it is right in front of you to prevent twisting your back.

2. Make sure you are in good alignment by centering your rib cage over your pelvis prior to bending over. (Do a **Baby Bod® Alignment Check** first.)

3. Start to bend over by doing the Bow, and then lift one leg and bend the knee you are standing on as you bend over to lift up the

4. Drop the leg you lifted as you return to standing.

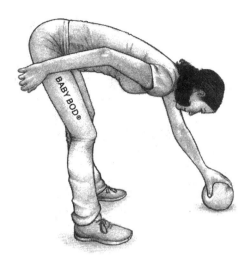

DON'T Do This:

Question: Can you see what's wrong with the way the woman in the illustration is bending?

Answer: The woman is bending in her back and not bending her knees.

She could reduce the strain on her back by using the Golfer's Lift or the Half-Kneel Lift on the next page.

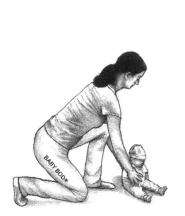
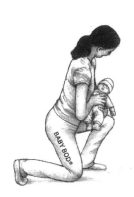
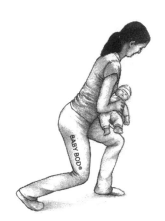
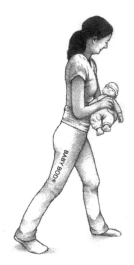

Half-Kneel Lift

1. To lift your child up off the floor, make sure to get close to your baby so you don't have to reach.

2. Get into a half-kneeling position. Kneel on one knee and bend the other leg at the knee and hip with your foot firmly planted on the ground.

3. Lift your baby with both arms and hold the baby close to the center of your body.

4. Make sure you are in good alignment, with your chest centered over your pelvis, before you start to stand up. (Do a **Baby Bod® Alignment Check**.)

5. To get up, EXHALE as you push the weight of your body upwards with your legs and slowly return to the standing position.

Lighten Up Your Handbag:

It is best to try to make your handbag as light as possible, so that it weighs no more than a pound or two. This is especially important if you have to carry your baby and your handbag while your body is still healing. Here's how to lighten what's in your bag:

1. Use a lightweight handbag made out of cloth and with very little hardware.

2. Use a lightweight wallet.

3. Remove anything that you don't absolutely need from your wallet, like change, extra credit cards, etc.

4. Try to use the calendar on your phone instead of carrying a separate calendar.

5. Ask yourself if you really need some of the items that can accumulate in your handbag. Here are good questions to pose to yourself:

    - *Do I really need to carry my make-up bag or brush? (Try to leave an extra make-up set and brush in your office for touch-ups.)*

    - *Do I really need to carry around several sets of keys, or just the ones for my front door and car?*

    - *Do I really need to carry around such a large bottle of water? Maybe just a few ounces will do.*

    - *Do I really need to carry around an umbrella today?*

Walking or Running with a Stroller

I hope you followed my advice in the last chapter and found a stroller that fits your body. That will make it easier to maintain correct alignment, which is something you want to check every now and then when you're pushing the stroller.

If you're going to be jogging with the stroller, I recommend that you wear supportive shorts or undergarments for several months after you deliver (see Chapters Eight and Nine for a list of external support garments). Otherwise, the repetitive jarring caused by running could contribute to pelvic organ prolapse and straining the pelvic floor and lower abdominal muscles. (Please consider waiting until you are able to pass the Straight Leg Raise Stability Test and the Jumping Test, found in Chapter Fifteen, before returning to a running program.)

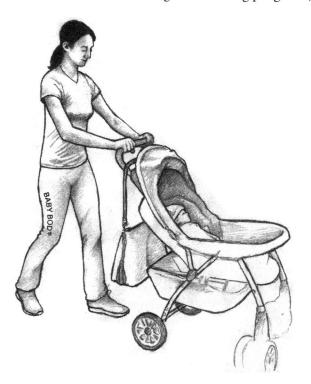

+ Stand close enough to the stroller so you don't have to reach forward with your arms. The distance you stand from the stroller may depend on your activity.

+ If you are walking, you need give yourself enough distance so that you can walk at your normal pace. Lean a little forward as you walk and keep your head aligned over your chest rather than jutting it forward.

+ **If you are jogging with a jogging stroller,** you will need to stand a little further away from the handlebars and lean your body forward to promote a good pace. Make sure you are close enough that you don't have to crane your neck forward. Try to keep your head aligned over your chest.

+ Don't lock your arms. Keep them slightly bent.

+ When you are holding the handlebars, keep your wrists straight.

+ Try to place your bags on the stroller instead of carrying them.

+ Try to bend forward at the hips and not by rounding out your back by using the Bow (as described in Chapter Fifteen.)

+ Don't "push" your stroller with your arms or upper body. Try to engage your entire body by leaning forward while you are walking or running.

+ Again, keep your alignment in mind. Keep your head, chest and pelvis aligned at all times. You might find it helpful to do a **Baby Bod® Alignment Check** every so often while you are walking and running.[A]

[A] Some of the information in this section first appeared in "Safe Strides: Jogging Stroller Safety Tips," which is an article I was interviewed for and appeared on the Fit4Mom blog. It can be accessed at *http://fit4mom.com/latest/blog/safe-strides-jogging-stroller-safety-tips.*

DON'T Do This:

Question: Can you find at least three things wrong in the illustration below?

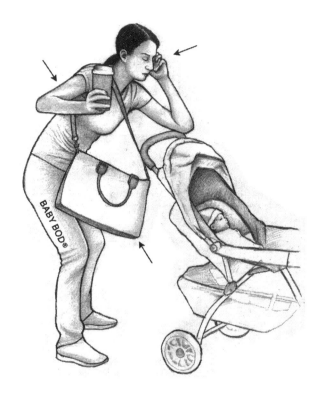

Answer: Mom is doing too much: talking on the phone, and carrying her handbag and a coffee while pushing the stroller. She is also too far away from the stroller and not using her arms to push the stroller.

Here's how to fix it: Hang the bag on stroller, get a cup attachment to carry your coffee or water, and don't talk on the phone while you are walking. Also, stand close enough to the stroller so you can easily push the stroller with your arms without bending in the back.

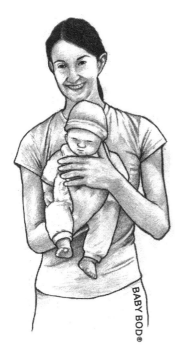

HOLDING YOUR BABY
Front Hold

It is best to hold your baby close to the center of your body.

Side Hold

If you do carry your baby on one side, try to hold the baby up and let his or her head rest on your shoulder. Make sure to alternate sides. If you continuously carry your baby on one side of your body, you risk straining your back, hips and neck.

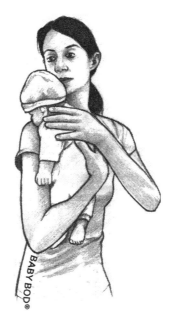

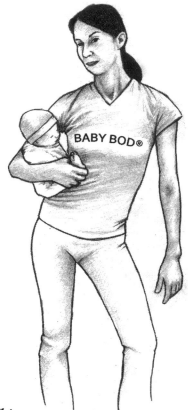

DON'T Do This:

Question: What is wrong with the woman's alignment in the illustration?

Answer: Mom is holding the baby on one hip and is forcing her pelvis to the side and out of good alignment. She is at risk of straining her back, hips and neck.

* * *

Practice these moves until you get to the point where you move correctly without having to think about it. Soon, you'll soon be getting your **Baby Bod**® on all day long! And you'll have a flat, sexy belly to show for it!

CHAPTER FIVE
Straight Leg Raise – Core Stability Test

PART 1: Straight Leg Raise (Without Compression)	No?	Yes?
Does one leg feel heavier than the other?		
Do you feel like your pelvis is rocking while doing a straight leg raise?		
Do you notice any pain (in the pelvis, abdomen or back)? If so, record where.		
Do you notice a bulging in the middle of your belly?		

PART 2: Straight Leg Raise (With Compression Hand or Belt)	No?	Yes?
Did one leg feel heavier than the other without the compression? And then feel lighter with the compression from your hands or the belt?		
Do you feel like your pelvis is rocking less?		
Do you notice that you have less pain? If so, record where the pain relief occurred (in the pelvis, abdomen or back).		
Do you notice less bulging in the middle of your belly?		

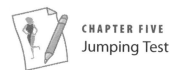

CHAPTER FIVE
Jumping Test

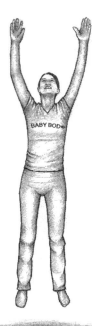

Jumping Test (Wait until 3 Months Postpartum. Nursing mothers may want to wait longer.)	No?	Yes?
Do you feel any pain? If so, record where (pelvis, pelvic floor, abdomen, or back).		
Does it feel like your internal organs are "bouncing" up and down against your pelvic floor?		
Did you have any leakage of urine, feces or gas?		
Do you notice a bulging in the middle of your belly?		

CHAPTER SIX

Check for Intra-Abdominal Pressure

The purpose of the first part of this test is to help you experience what intra-abdominal pressure feels like. The second part will help you experience what it feels like when you exhale and decrease the pressure.

Part 1: Place a hand on your tummy, take a big breath in, and hold it. Do you feel your abdominal muscles stretching and your belly popping outwards?
☐ Yes ☐ No

Part 2: Exhale. Then place a hand on your belly and gently exhale, as if you are cleaning a pair of sunglasses. Make sure to empty all the air in your lungs. When you finish exhaling, do you feel as if your abdominal muscles are working more and pulling in your tummy a bit?
☐ Yes ☐ No

Next: Do the assessment below. The point of this chart is to help you become aware of when you hold your breath during exertion:

Do You Hold Your Breath When You Do The Following?	No?	Yes?
Pick up or carry your baby?		
Pick up heavy packages or the stroller?		
Reach for something on the top shelf in the grocery store?		
Push a vacuum or heavy door?		
Lift a pot of pasta off the stove?		
Pull something heavy?		
Play sports like tennis, especially when you hit the ball?		

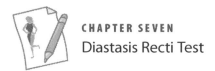

CHAPTER SEVEN
Diastasis Recti Test

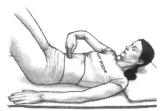

Diastasis Recti	Your Answers
Do you feel a soft spot between your muscles?	
How many fingers can you fit into the soft spot? Is it one finger width? Two fingers' width? Three fingers' width?	
Feel for the separation about 2 inches above the belly button. Write down how far apart it is:	
Feel for the separation about 1 inch below the belly button. Write down how far apart it is:	

Incontinence

Incontinence Questions – What Are You Experiencing?	No?	Yes?
1. Do you leak pee when you cough, sneeze, run or pick up a grocery package?		
2. Can you hold your urine for 2 ½ hours?		
3. Are you able to urinate with an uninterrupted flow? Or does your flow stop and go?		
4. Do you find yourself making several toilet stops per day, "just in case" you need to go later? Or do you think you have a "tiny bladder"?		
5. Do you always make it to the bathroom on time?		
6. Do you feel any pain or discomfort, like burning, when you pee?		
7. Do you find you have to return to use the toilet moments after you thought you had finished urinating?		
8. Do you need to use pads to prevent urine "spillage" onto your clothing? If so, how many pads per day?		

Pelvic Organ Prolapse

Pelvic Organ Prolapse Questions	No?	Yes?
Do you feel as if there's "something" in your vagina?		
Do you feel as if something seems to be coming out of or pushing down on your pelvic floor every time you cough, sneeze, or jump?		
Can you feel something coming out of your vagina, especially after passing a bowel movement?		
When you urinate, are you able to fully empty your bladder?		
Do you leak urine, or have a constant "dribble" of urine leaking from your bladder?		
Do you have a constant urge to urinate?		
Do you have to return to the toilet to empty your bladder shortly after you urinate?		
Are you able to fully empty your bowels at one time, or do you need to return frequently to finish making a bowel movement?		

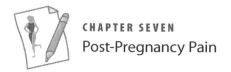

Post-Pregnancy Pain

Pain After Childbirth	Yes? Give a Brief Description	No?
On a Scale of 1 to 10 with 10 being the worst, how would you rate your pain?		
What makes the pain worse?		
What makes the pain better?		
Is it worse in the morning, afternoon or evening?		
Does the pain interfere with sleeping?		
Do you feel it when you're getting up from sitting down?		
Or when you're sitting?		
Or when you're walking?		
Or going up a set of stairs?		
Or when you are passing a bowel movement or urinating?		
Is it interfering with your life, with your normal everyday activities?		
How much can you walk without pain?		
What activity causes the most pain?		
Does the pain prevent you from exercising?		

CHAPTER ELEVEN

How to Identify Your Alignment Dysfunction

Once you have the picture of yourself, please take a close look at the curves in your back and how you hold your body. What do you see? Do you have any of the alignment dysfunctions below? Try to recheck your progress on a monthly basis.

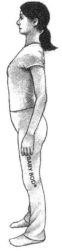

Mid-Back Clenching (Military Posture)

☐ Is your upper chest wall leaning backwards?

Mid-Back Clencher

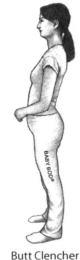

Butt Clenching

☐ Do you squeeze your buttocks tightly?

Butt Clencher

Living on a Cliff

☐ Are you using a mix of both Mid-Back Clenching and Butt Clenching?

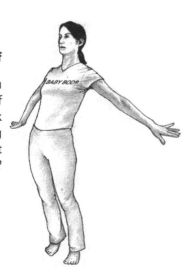

Living on a Cliff

Chest Collapser

☐ Do you stand with your chest collapsed with your neck and pelvis pushed forward?

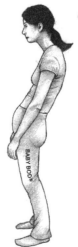

Chest Collasper

CHAPTER FOURTEEN
Cough Test

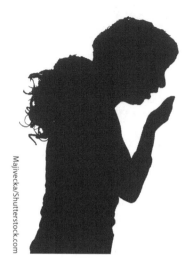

Majivecka/Shutterstock.com

I would like you to stand and cough. What did you feel going on in your bottom? Did you feel as if your pelvic floor dropped downwards? OK, that is normal.
☐ Yes

Now I would like you to contract your pelvic floor muscles by doing the Pelvic-Core Starter and holding it. Now COUGH. Did you feel your pelvic floor drop less?
☐ Yes?

The point of this is to make you aware of how much more support you can offer your body when you actively do a pelvic floor muscle contraction. Try to remember to *contract your pelvic floor* **prior** *to coughing, sneezing and laughing. And when exerting yourself*, like picking up a laundry basket, heavy bag or even when you get up from a chair.

BABY BOD® EXERCISE TRACKER

This chart was designed to help you track your exercises as you perform them. For more detail information on how to do the exercises please refer to the directions in the book.

Instead of using this chart, you may download the **Baby Bod Exercise Tracker App** which is available on iTunes or Google Play.

PRELIMINARY BABY BOD® PROGRAM		☑ CHECK						
Baby Bod® Alignment Check	**Reps / Times per Day**	S	M	T	W	T	F	S
• Neutral Pelvis Position • Straighten Up Spine • Stack Chest Over Pelvis • Shoulder Rolls • Chin Tucks • Pelvic Floor Contraction	Do as a series several times a day—ideally, once an hour.							
Neutral Pelvis Position 	Do this about 5 times and stop when you are in the mid-range. *Precaution: If you had a C-section, only do this in pain free ranges. If you feel pain or pulling in your incision, decrease the range you are moving or wait until after your six-week checkup before doing this part of the Alignment Check.*							
Straighten Up Spine 	Do this 1 time to reposition your spine.							
Stack Chest Over Pelvis 	Do this 1 time to reposition your chest over your pelvis.							

PRELIMINARY BABY BOD® PROGRAM   ☑ CHECK

Baby Bod® Alignment Check	Reps / Times per Day	S	M	T	W	T	F	S
Shoulder Rolls	Do this 1 time to reposition your shoulders.							
Chin Tuck	Do this 1 time to reposition your head over your chest.							
Pelvic Floor Contraction	Do 1 gentle pelvic floor contraction and then release it.							
Breathing Exercises	**Reps / Times per Day**	S	M	T	W	T	F	S
Lower Tummy Breathing	Do for 2-3 minutes / 1-2x's per day. Alternate positions: Lying on back, sitting and standing.							

PRELIMINARY BABY BOD® PROGRAM   ☑ CHECK

Breathing Exercises	Reps / Times per Day	S	M	T	W	T	F	S
Rib Expanders	Do for 2-3 minutes / 1-2x's per day. Alternate positions: Lying on back, sitting and standing.							

Warm Up Exercises	Reps / Times per Day	S	M	T	W	T	F	S

• Head Bobble
• Chin Tucks
• Shoulder Roll
• Upper Back Stretch
• Bali Dancer
• Trunk Twister
• Pelvic Rock Series
  — Pelvic Up and Downs
  — Pelvic Circles
  — Pelvic Tilts
	Done in a Series (one after the other)							

Head Bobble	Do 5 times to each side.							
Chin Tuck	Do this 1 time to reposition your head over your chest.							

PRELIMINARY BABY BOD® PROGRAM   ☑ CHECK

Warm Up Exercises	Reps / Times per Day	S	M	T	W	T	F	S
Shoulder Roll	Do 5 times.							
Upper back Stretch	Do 5 times. *Precaution: If you had a C-section, start after six-week check.*							
Bali Dancer	Move wrist up and down 10 times. Do 2 times a day.							
Trunk Twister	Do 2-3 to each side. *Precaution: If you had a C-section, start after six-week check.*							

PRELIMINARY BABY BOD® PROGRAM		☑ CHECK						
Warm Up Exercises	**Reps / Times per Day**	**S**	**M**	**T**	**W**	**T**	**F**	**S**
Pelvic Rock Series — Pelvic Up and Down	Do 5 times in each direction. *Precaution: If you had a C-section, only do this in pain free ranges. If you feel pain or pulling in your incision, decrease the range you are moving or wait until after your six-week checkup before* doing this part of the warm up exercises.							
Pelvic Rock Series — Pelvic Circles								
Pelvic Rock Series — Pelvic Tilt	Do 5 times in each direction. *Precaution: If you had a C-section, only do this in pain free ranges. If you feel pain or pulling in your incision, decrease the range you are moving or wait until after your six-week checkup before* doing this part of the warm up exercises.							

PRELIMINARY BABY BOD® PROGRAM			☑ CHECK						
Walking Program	**Reps / Times per Day**	**S**	**M**	**T**	**W**	**T**	**F**	**S**	
Daily Walking	Start with 10-minute mini-walks a few times a day. Build up to one 30-minute daily walk. (On the days you cannot fit in a 30-minute walk, make sure to fit in a few mini-10-minute walks.)								
Pelvic Core Starter	**Reps / Times per Day**	**S**	**M**	**T**	**W**	**T**	**F**	**S**	
Pelvic Core Starter*	Hold contraction for 3 seconds, then 3 quick flicks. Rest for 6 seconds. Repeat series 10 times / 3x's a day. Alternate positions: Lying on back, sitting and standing. *Precaution: If you have a Grade 3 or 4 tear, do not start this exercise until after your six-week check and have medical clearance to exercise.*								

* After a week, progress these by holding for 4 seconds, then 4 quick flicks. Rest for 8 seconds. Repeat series 10 times / 3x's a day.

* After two weeks, continue progressing by holding for 5 seconds. Then do 5 quick flicks, and then rest for 10 seconds. Repeat series 10 times / 3x's a day.

Start the Advanced Baby Bod® Exercise Program after you have completed 1 week of the Preliminary Baby Bod®

ADVANCED BABY BOD® PROGRAM	☑ CHECK							
Preliminary Program	**Reps / Times per Day**	S	M	T	W	T	F	S
Refer to prior chart for a detailed list and illustrations.								
Baby Bod® Alignment Check	Do daily (once an hour).							
Breathing Exercises Lower Tummy Rib Expanders	Do daily.							
Warm Ups	Do daily.							
Walking Program	Daily 30-minute walks (do 2-3 mini-10-minute walks on off days). You can skip walking on the days you use cardio equipment to work out.							
Pelvic Core Starters * Alternate positions	After doing these for 1-week, progress these by holding for 4 seconds, then 4 quick flicks. Rest for 8 seconds. Repeat series 10 times / 3x's a day. After two weeks, continue progressing by holding for 5 seconds. Then do 5 quick flicks, and then rest for 10 seconds. Repeat series 10 times / 3x's a day.							

* If you are just starting the Pelvic Core Starter because you had a 3rd or 4th degree tear, start with 3-second holds and 3 quick contractions and progress to 5-second holds over a 2-week period).

ADVANCED BABY BOD® PROGRAM   ☑ CHECK

Kicker Starters	Reps / Times per Day	S	M	T	W	T	F	S
The Bow	5 times standing.							
The Stork	Hold for 10 seconds. Do 3 times on each leg.							

Strengthening Exercises	Reps / Times per Day	S	M	T	W	T	F	S
The Bridge	Hold for 5 seconds, and then pulse 5 times. Do 5 times.							
Heel Tapping / Slides	Repeat 10 times on each side. Progress to Heel Slides							
Side Leg Glides	Do 15 times with each leg.							

ADVANCED BABY BOD® PROGRAM		☑ CHECK						
Strengthening Exercises	**Reps / Times per Day**	**S**	**M**	**T**	**W**	**T**	**F**	**S**
Leg Circles	Do 10 clockwise and 10 counterclockwise circles.							
Underneath Side leg Lift	Do 20 times with each leg.							
Knee Touch Down	Do 10 times with each leg.							
Table Top – Rib Expanders	Hold for 15 seconds and repeat 2 times. Gradually build up to holding 30 seconds and repeat 2 times.							
Side Planks	Hold for 15 seconds and repeat 2 times. Gradually build up to holding 30 seconds and repeat 2 times.							

Strengthening Exercises continue on next page.

ADVANCED BABY BOD® PROGRAM   ☑ CHECK

Strengthening Exercises	Reps / Times per Day	S	M	T	W	T	F	S
Butt Lifter	Hold for 5 seconds, and then pulse 5 times. Do 5 times on each leg.							
Chair Squats / Standing Squats	Do 10 times. Progress to doing it without chair.							
Salt Water Taffy Pulls Chair / Standing	Do 15 times to each side with resistance band. Progress to doing it in standing.							
Walking Program	**Reps / Times per Day**	**S**	**M**	**T**	**W**	**T**	**F**	**S**
Daily Walking	Try to do daily 30-minute walks, on the off days try to fit in three mini-10-minute walks.							

HOW TO FIND A PHYSICAL THERAPIST IN YOUR AREA

You can find a women's health physical therapist or physiotherapist who has a practice in your area by going on the world wide web. Here are websites that can help:[A]

United States

American Physical Therapy Association: http://www.MoveForwardPT or www.apta.org/findapt

To find a pelvic physical therapist: http://www.womenshealthapta.org

United Kingdom

Charted Society of Physiotherapists: http://www.csp.org.uk

Ireland

The Irish Society of Chartered Physiotherapists: http://www.iscp.ie

Canada

Canadian Physiotherapy Association: http://www.physiotherapy.ca

To find a pelvic physiotherapist, look up the Women's Health Division on the website.

Australia

Australian Physiotherapy Association: http://www.physiotherapy.asn.au

To find a pelvic physiotherapist, look up the Continence and Women's Health section on the website.

[A] (Note: This list is limited. If your country is not included in this list, look up the national organization for physical therapists or physiotherapists in your area.)

Made in the USA
Middletown, DE
21 September 2021